Dude, You Don't Have to be Fat

Eat great. Lose weight. Live well.
(Yeah, it really is that simple.)

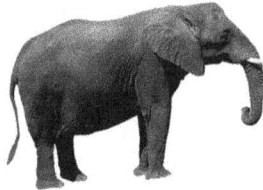

Mike Nappa
with Edwin Risenhoover, MD

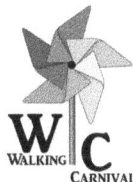

W C
WALKING
CARNIVAL

Dude, You Don't Have to be Fat
ISBN 978-1-939953-07-0

Published by Walking Carnival Books
an imprint of Nappaland Communications Inc.
1674 East 29th Street
Loveland, CO 80537

"Elephant" image used courtesy of Microsoft Design Gallery.

Disclaimer:
This book is a general guide only and should never substitute for the medical care and health supervision of a qualified medical professional. The research, nutrition principles, experience, and facts presented in this publication are accurate to the best of the authors' knowledge. However, this book is intended as an informational resource and should never be used as a substitute or replacement for the care, diagnosis, and/or treatment prescribed by a licensed physician or nutritionist. The authors and the publisher are not responsible for any adverse effects or consequences resulting from the use of information in this book. The authors encourage the reader to seek out the opinion of a personal physician before using the information in this book, and/or in conjunction with the use of this material. It is the responsibility of the reader to consult with a physician or other qualified health care professional in regard to the reader's personal health.

www.WalkingCarnival.com
www.Nappaland.com

1 2 3 4 5 6 7 •• 2020 2019 2018 2017

"Make Readers Happy"

"**Dude, You Don't Have to be Fat** *is ideal for men everywhere. There's not much help out there to inspire us guys to cook, to eat well at home, and to make smart choices when we eat out. Mike Nappa gives us the right tools to make the right choices so we can love what we eat—and look good eating it too. This book allows us 'dudes' to start a lifestyle of healthy eating (not a diet!), and to stay on the plan without coming off. Great stuff!"*

TV Chef Daniel Green
Judge on Food Network's Kitchen Inferno, *On-Air TV Host, Evine Live and Popular culinary author* (Healthy Dining for Life; Healthy Eating for Lower Cholesterol)

*****

"*Healthy eating and making good lifestyle choices seem be more difficult for my male patients. I would highly recommend* **Dude, You Don't Have to be Fat** *to all men who want to take control of their lifestyle, and improve their overall wellness, through healthy eating.*"

Dr. Kim Bruno
Certified Clinical Nutritionist

*****

"*Obesity is epidemic in the United States and is directly related to medical conditions such as hypertension and Diabetes. It is drastically altering the health of the American populace. Mike Nappa's book* **Dude, You Don't Have to be Fat**, *is written in a highly readable format and provides a logical, easy method of dietary control which, if followed, would substantially improve the incidence of obesity in the US. I highly recommend it to anyone truly interested in improving their current health and lessening their risk of future heart attacks or strokes.*"

Thomas P. Kasenberg
Doctor of Osteopathy

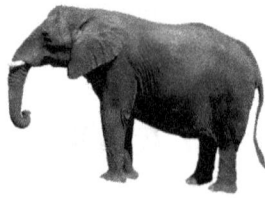

Table of Contents

Introduction:
The Rules

Rule #1: A man should never be hungry.

Okay, there are exceptions to that rule. Like poverty. Or being stranded in the Arctic after your plane has crash-landed. Or maybe when your mother-in-law serves cranberry-raisin meatloaf and pinto bean pie.

But generally speaking, if you're an American with a job, living in this country where food is abundant and comparatively cheap, you should never have to go hungry in order to look good for your favorite girl. So forget all that garbage about "portion control" and gimmicky starvation diets and anything else that says you can't have a great body unless your stomach is growling all the time.

Remember Rule #1:

You should *never* have to go hungry.

Got it? Okay, on to...

Rule #2: Food is not your enemy.

And yes, this applies to your refrigerator and restaurants and fast-food joints and anyplace else you grub food. Truth is, you are your only enemy when it comes to living a healthy, enjoyable lifestyle.

Too many guys feel powerless to control what and how they eat. They assume that since Funyuns exist, they must be swallowed. That it's a man's responsibility to happily suck up whatever is set before him. That it's a sign of weakness to read a Nutrition Facts label or ask a waitress to put the sauce on the side. That a kitchen is some mysterious enemy that can only be overcome by staying out of it, or devouring everything in it.

Crockhockets.

Take control of your own life, Dude.

Don't blame your kitchen or your girlfriend's cooking or the chef at Applebee's for the fact that you can't see your boxers anymore when you look down. You are responsible for yourself—that includes what you eat and the way your body looks and feels.

We'll dig into that more, later.

Why Alaska's part of the United States:

"Canadians went in there, saw [the Eskimos] eating blubber and said, "Huh, the Americans already got here."
—Jim Gaffigan [1]

Rule #3: Eat great. Lose weight. Live well.

Hey, Rule #3 is the reason you want this book. It's the difference between a long, happy life and a short, fatty one. It's the key to feeling good about yourself—and looking even better. It's the catalyst for joy, love, companionship, and satisfaction in your everyday existence.

If you eat well, you can lose weight and live well because your body will *be* well.

Understood? Good.

Now let's get down to business.

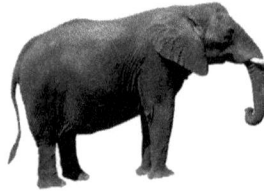

How To Use This Book

Basic fact:
Your refrigerator is your first ally in
taking charge of your health life.

Learn how to manage that common kitchen appliance, and the "fridge benefits" you receive—better health, more energy, better relationships with friends and family, higher confidence, and more—will change forever the way you look at yourself. Literally.

Your second ally is this book, which I've titled *Dude, You Don't Have to be Fat*. Let that title be your constant reminder that the key to your health and eating satisfaction lies always within your reach.

So what can you expect from *Dude, You Don't Have to be Fat*? A lot. By using this book, you'll:

• Take charge of your own body—and see the difference in your mirror.
• Learn how to get "fridge benefits" anyplace you eat—at home, at a restaurant, at a fast-food place, or even at a friend's house for dinner.
• Discover a simple approach to eating well—and loving it.
• Enjoy your food—without letting it harm you.
• Feel better about yourself, your body, your life, and your future.
• Discover easy ways to make your refrigerator an ally instead of your enemy.
• Get off the fad diet and get-skinny-quick treadmills.
• Become smarter, healthier, and more confident.
• Love your lifestyle—and live longer to boot.

However, I want to make one thing clear. This is a book about achieving "food health" for an average guy. It's not about how to turn yourself into a yoked, steroid-packed, muscle-bound stud.

Check out my picture on the back cover. Sure, for my age I'm a good-looking hombre (yes, I'm a lot older than you are; get over it.). And yes, I managed to marry a hot wife—and keep her happy for 25+ years. (No, she's not in the picture, but a guy's got to brag every once in awhile, right?)

But I think it's obvious I'm not going to star in the Olympics or pull down millions in the NFL anytime soon. In fact, I live with a chronic illness that pretty much prevents me from pursuing dreams of athletic fortune and fame. That's okay. I'm likely to outlive most Olympians and pro athletes anyway. I'm not abusing my body today in the pursuit of brief athletic glory that'll fade tomorrow and leave me worse for the wear for the rest of my life.

I'm good with that.

My guess is that you're not a pro athlete either. You might even be someone like me who suffers from a chronic illness, or maybe you have a physical disability that limits how much you can realistically exercise. That's okay. You don't have to be a baller or a workout warrior or a gym rat to maintain a healthy body and a satisfying lifestyle in your youth, middle age, and old age. Anybody who tells you that you do is just selling advertising.

Yes, regular exercise is good for your health, and yes, if you can, you'd be wise to live an active lifestyle to go along with the smart eating advice you'll find in this book. In fact, my co-author for this book, Dr. Edwin Risenhoover, is an avid cyclist—and that definitely contributes to his continued good health. I'd love it if you did something like that (and so would your wife). And yes, if you want to pursue a career as a mixed martial arts champion or something, you'll probably want to join a gym and develop a high-impact fitness regimen as well. But you don't have to—and I'm living proof.

Of course, you don't have to believe just me. A recent study on weight loss and health revealed that diet alone (i.e., what you eat and swallow) controls 75 percent of your weight status. [2] That means, as Dr. Kim Bruno explains, "You really can control your health by the food you choose to put in your mouth." [3]

So, yes, exercise is definitely important and you should do it if you can. But this book will focus on that other 75 percent of your body maintenance, helping you become a pro at food health so you can experience all the benefits that go with that.

Besides, if you want to be a mixed martial arts champion, I'm probably not writing this book for you anyway. (But good luck—I'm rooting for you!) I'm writing *Dude, You Don't Have to be Fat* for regular guys like me. Guys who think about going to the gym, but almost never get there. Guys who want to see their wives smile at the sight of them. Men who want to enjoy a good meal without feeling guilty or worried about their health or ashamed about it later. Guys who want to look good, and feel good, each day of a normal life:

- On the subway headed to work.
- Sitting in a pew on Sunday morning.
- In the coffee bar.
- Taking your best girl to the movies.
- Watching a football game with friends and family.
- Playing with your kids after work.
- Fixing up the house on the weekend.
- Chatting with the neighbors about the weather.
- Attending your daughter's dance recital.
- Cheering at your son's soccer game.
- Going dancing Saturday night.
- Even just sitting around watching American Idol with your family.

I want guys like us to become so comfortable with our bodies, that we don't even notice them anymore. We just assume we look good, because we feel good. That's what *Dude, You Don't Have to be Fat* is all about. So if you're a guy like that, then keep reading.

Is This a New Diet?

Now this is important: No.

Dude, You Don't Have to be Fat isn't a quick fix. It's not some short-term diet for you to try on for awhile and then abandon six months from now. If that's your goal, put down this book right now, cuz you're wasting my time. And you're being kind of stupid and desperate with your own life, and I'd rather not be involved in that. I'll wait until you're ready for a real change to happen.

This isn't a fad or a quick-change gimmick or get-skinny-in-a-month scheme. When you embrace the *Dude, You Don't Have to be Fat* lifestyle you embrace it from today to forever—and (believe it or not), it won't be long until you won't want to go back to eating the junk you used to consume.

Anything Else We Should Know?

While we're at it, let's clarify a few other things that *Dude, You Don't Have to be Fat* is not:

• *It's not punishment* for being out of shape physically, mentally, or spiritually. It's actually a reward. When we don't take charge of our own bodies, that's when we're truly punishing ourselves. Instead, DYDHtbF puts you in control—and brings you the reward of a satisfying, healthy lifestyle.

• *It's not a chore to be tolerated or endured.* Leave behind the idea that eating well means a lifetime of boring and tasteless food. That's just propaganda from people who are too lazy to attempt what you're about to accomplish. Instead, think of this lifestyle change as an adventure where you may not even know what wonderful surprises will be revealed as you round each corner.

• *It's not a long list of "no-no's."* Seriously, no guy among us wants to always be saying, "I can't eat that, I can't drink that..." We want to be saying "I can have it all!" With the *Dude, You Don't Have to be Fat* lifestyle you'll find yourself saying "yes" more than ever. Yes to good eating. Yes to body nutrition. Yes to peace of mind. Yes to satisfaction. And more. Sound too good to be true? Well, give it a try and you can be the judge of that. (You already know how I feel about it.)

• *It's not a confusing, hard-to-follow approach.* This entire book is based on one simple idea: lower fat = higher satisfaction. That means you can forget about counting calories or adding up Weight Watcher's points or drinking Metamucil with your meals. All you have to do is be aware of how much fat you're eating in a day—and this book will help make that easy for you.

My Story

All right, we're just about ready. And now that you and I are becoming friends, I think it'd be good if I were to finish this chapter by telling you my story, so you can understand better where I'm coming from and why I wrote this book.

I was 36 years old and, after surviving a scare from the aftereffects of a wicked gallbladder surgery, I thought I was in pretty good health. My kid was in elementary school. My wife (beautiful as ever) was pursuing her own career in writing and editing. I was a professional writer and editor, a small businessman, and a generally doing fine.

At 5'11" and weighing in at about 210, I figured I could lose a little weight, but I wasn't too worried about it. After all, I was leading a moderately active, enjoyable life, and managing to keep up (sort of) with my energetic 10-year-old. Most importantly, my wife wasn't complaining. (Whew!) No problems, right?

Well, wrong.

After a routine blood test for an insurance examination, I got an urgent call from my doctor. He insisted that I come in for more tests. "There's cause for concern," he said when we met afterward. "Your tests confirm heavy fatty deposits on your liver."

My liver was overweight? What?

"That means your liver is engorged with fat, along with other organs inside you, and that affects the way your body works. If you don't do something about this now, you'll develop heart disease, or liver disease, or diabetes, or any combination of these within the next 10 years."

"But I feel fine," I said.

"And you look fine," he said. "You're not obese. You carry your weight well. But that doesn't change what's going on inside your body." He paused while I tried to take it all in. Then he said, "Your son deserves to have his father around for a long time. For that to happen, you'll need to make a change."

He gave me some literature, recommended a few books, and sent me on my way.

I was dumbstruck. My wife and son were away visiting relatives, and I was actually glad to have the house to myself.

I have to change the way I eat. Today. Forever.

That thought was so overwhelming, I immediately tore open a prepackaged Little Debbie brownie with fudgy-chocolate icing and shoved it down my mouth.

I looked at the plastic wrapper in my hands and thought, *Fat on my liver is literally killing me from the inside out.*

Finally, I called my wife and we talked about the doctor's diagnosis. By the time she got home a few days later, I'd read everything I could get my hands on about reducing fat in daily eating. It was still a little overwhelming, but now at least I knew that it could be done. We went to the grocery store and began reading labels—and it was an eye-opening experience! We were both surprised to learn how much fat we'd been unwittingly chowing day after day. And we were ready to do something about it.

From that day forward, our refrigerator became our greatest ally in the pursuit of eating well—and loving it. We'd finally discovered that our kitchen had "fridge benefits" that could keep us healthy without sacrificing the joy of a good bite to eat. That little discovery changed everything.

Fast-forward to today. As I write this book, my weight has leveled off to around 175-180 pounds—and stayed that way for years. My liver has completely reversed its prior damaged state and now functions in perfect health—thank God! I'm no longer at increased risk for heart disease, liver disease, or diabetes. Not long ago I had an annual checkup, and my doctor said to me, "You have the body of a much younger man. You'll probably outlive us all."

What's more, I eat great-tasting food every single day. I eat when I'm hungry, and I eat until I'm full. I've managed to stick around long enough to see my son grow into a fine young man and marry a fine young woman. (Way to go, kid!)

Each day my body functions well, enabling me to pursue my life passions without the hindrance of unnecessary (and unwanted) health problems added to my chronic illness.

So, that's my story and I'm sticking with it. Why? Because it works—and I'm living proof. Now, if you're ready to reap some those same kinds of "fridge benefits" in your own life, then turn the page to Part 1 of this book, and let's get started.

Part 1

Getting Started

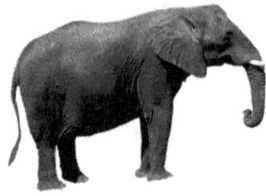

One:
Why Eat Well?

When we got the news that I had to significantly lower the amount of fat I ate, I had to make the change immediately.

There was no "grace period" for reversing the damaging effects that decades of fat consumption had wreaked on my body.

My wife, Amy, and I grabbed as many books and articles as we could to learn about how to fill my body with what it needed. Interestingly enough, the more we read about the changes I had to make, the more Amy also wanted to make changes in the way she was eating. We both were quickly learning how much fat we were dumping into our bodies—and we wanted to stop. But how?

It's one thing to optimistically say, "I'm going to change my lifestyle!" It's quite another thing to actually do it. Because I have a chronic illness, I'm also limited in the amount of physical activity and exercise I can do. (Long story short: If my body heat gets too high for too long, it triggers nausea and vomiting—a complication left over from that wicked gallbladder surgery I told you about previously.) So I had to approach this idea of healthy eating realistically.

Here's what my wife and I learned.

Just the Facts

The key to getting the most benefit from your eating habits, I discovered, is to maintain a discipline of eating lower-fat foods. And that's the central premise for *Dude, You Don't Have to be Fat.*

Like I said before, I've learned through personal experience that low-fat eating yields higher satisfaction in health and life. Now, you could just take my word for that and skip on to the next chapter if you like. But if you've got a few minutes, let's go ahead and talk about why that's true, about some real, tangible benefits that come from taking a low-fat approach to the way you live your life.

After all, why should you even want to change the way you eat? What are the benefits of low-fat eating?

Now—and this is important—I'm not a doctor or a professional nutritionist. I'm just an average guy like you. Yet it's been easy for me to research the benefits of cutting down on fatty food habits, as there are stacks and stacks of books, articles, and studies on the importance of low-fat eating.

I also recruited my good friend Dr. Edwin Risenhoover to help me deliver medically-sound, practical information for you in this book. Eddie is a licensed family physician with two decades of experience practicing medicine. Even better, he's been by my side as I worked through the everyday *Dude, You Don't Have to be Fat* lifestyle over the past decade—and he's seen it work firsthand.

Now, Eddie and I won't go into all the specific medical studies and statistical data here about how a low-fat approach to eating has been tested and confirmed as a life-changer in regard to your health. But if you're really interested, you can check out some of the Recommended Resources listed at the end of this book (page 150) for more information on that. For now, let's just focus on the well-known facts:

No More Dieting

The first fridge benefit of changing to a lower-fat eating style is that it's *not* a diet.

When we say we're "on a diet," we tend to think of our changed eating habits as temporary. We think we'll count calories or eat only certain foods until we've achieved our ideal weight—then we can go back to our old eating habits again.

A sporadic diet like this actually means we're more likely to gain weight again—and become even more discouraged than before. So one of the first steps toward reaping the benefits of low-fat eating is this: Forget the idea of being on a diet.

Instead, determine to cheerfully say, "I'm permanently changing my lifestyle." No more "diet" means no more reason for the up-and-down roller coaster of weight loss and subsequent gain cycle.

It's the old "Tortoise and the Hare" philosophy. Instead of following fad diet "rabbits" that take off fast, then stall before finishing dead-last in the race, this lifestyle chooses the slow-and-steady tortoise approach. Day in, day out, we do the little things, choosing to fill ourselves with health until we don't need, or even want, unhealthy foods. We take one step at a time, shunning diets and living the lifestyle instead. Before long, like that victorious slowpoke of a turtle, we too will cross that finish line in first place—and be empowered by healthy habits to keep finishing first in the race of life.

No More Hunger Games

Let's face it, fellas. If you're like me, when it comes to eating and food health, your biggest fear is not a fat gut, or even being repulsive to women. It's being hungry. And we associate "eating healthy" with a constant, dissatisfied gnawing in the stomach. That kind of portion control "hunger game," found in so many deprivation diets, is simply a non-starter for me—and I'm betting it's a no-go for you as well.

Hey look, I grew up dirt poor. I know what it's like to be hungry simply because there's no money to buy food. I know what it's like to smell bacon and honestly think about breaking into somebody's home just to get it. And yes, I admit to stealing food from time to time when I was a kid, just to get my stomach to stop screaming. But, as I said before, if you're an American man with a job, there really is no reason for you to be hungry. Eating good food and maintaining a healthy body are not mutually exclusive.

I like the way Dr. Kim Bruno explains it. A certified clinical nutritionist, she reveals that eating "fast food, crappy food, quick food, processed food," actually leaves you feeling hungrier because it causes a quick increase, and then rapid decrease, in your glucose level. That, in turn, leaves you with a "kind of ravenous feeling of being really hungry." How to avoid that? "You want to eat foods that will sustain you longer." [4] Foods that don't leave you feeling hungry and craving more. Foods that truly satisfy—and taste great. That, my friend, is the way *Dude, You Don't Have to be Fat* works—and it's awesome. You really can live out Rule #1 in your life: A man should never be hungry.

Weight Loss

The most obvious benefit of a low-fat habit is weight loss.

The goal for eating less fat is truly to have better health—from your insides out. But a side benefit of choosing to fill your plate with healthful foods is that you'll start dropping unwanted pounds. This is not a gimmicky "lose 10 pounds in 10 days!" promise—and, in fact, your weight loss will likely move at a slower pace than what many of the fad diets out there promise. But that's okay, because your weight loss will happen at a slow, steady, natural pace. What physiologists know that most guys like us don't is that the body can really only lose about three pounds of fat in a week, maximum. If you drop more weight than that, it's usually just water weight that fluctuates depending on your hydration patterns. [5]

With *Dude, You Don't Have to be Fat*, you'll see weight loss happen gradually, but significantly, over several months. And you'll be able to keep off the pounds once you reach your body's natural, comfortable weight level because you lost it in a natural, permanent way.

Now, this is not to condemn people who are overweight. Some folks tell me, "I'm heavy, and I'm at peace with that." Well, God and our mamas do love us all, no matter how thick or thin we are. If you say that you're happy being overweight, then God bless ya li'l overworked heart. You can put down this book now on move on happily with your chosen life.

But...

I suspect that's not how you really feel. After all, you picked up this book, and you must have done it for a reason. And honestly, you can't ignore that being overweight is hard on any man's body—including yours.

For instance, carrying around extra pounds strains our muscles, bones, and internal organs in many ways. When we lighten the load our bodies carry, we help our bodies to perform at their peak—and that's what happens as a by-product of this kind of lifestyle change.

Fact is, I dropped 25 pounds during the first six months after switching to a low-fat eating style. And after about a year, I reached my body's ideal weight (around 175-180 pounds). What's more, this fat-reducing lifestyle has enabled me to keep those pounds off for more than a decade. Using only the *Dude, You Don't Have to be Fat* approach to eating, I've been able to maintain a consistent weight that looks good—and feels good. And you can too.

More Energy

Lowering your daily fat intake will also give you more energy.

Because I have a chronic health condition, for several years I was wary about volunteering or participating in some high-energy activities. There were too many days I simply didn't feel like I had the strength or that I could count on my body to cooperate. But within four months of cutting my fat intake, I was coaching my son's elementary school basketball team! Even with my chronic illness, eating less fat had improved my energy level.

Of course, that's just common sense if you think about it.

That 25+ pounds I lost initially is about as much as my preschool niece weighs. Now, honestly, it's no big deal for me to carry little Anika around on my shoulders for a while. Still, after only one hour of carrying her everywhere, I have to admit I get tired.

Now imagine what it would be like if I had to carry that little girl around all the time—that every time I stood up, she was on my shoulders; that every time I sat down, Ani was hanging onto my neck; that every time I walked around the mall I had to carry Anika's weight draped across my stomach. No wonder I was tired from being overweight! You would be too. In fact, if you're 25 pounds overweight, you probably are still tired.

Next, imagine the difference if, after years of carrying the weight of this little girl with me wherever I went, I suddenly discovered that Anika could walk on her own. What if I set her down and let her stroll beside me instead of bearing her weight myself? I'd feel the difference right away. I'd have more energy, and less pain and exhaustion.

That's what happened for me. And it will happen for you after a low-fat approach to eating prompts your body to lose weight too.

Better Career Prospects

Okay, yes, this is totally unfair, but the awful truth is that your weight affects how successful (or unsuccessful) you are in our image-conscious, American society. Whether you like it or not, you are judged in the workplace, at least in part, by your size.

Reader's Digest recently interviewed eighteen Human Resources professionals to find out the "secrets" these folks generally keep to themselves when hiring. You shouldn't be surprised to hear former HR executive, Suzanne Lucas, say it plainly, "Is it harder to get a job if you're fat?" she says. "Absolutely. Like George Clooney's character said in *Up in the Air*, 'I stereotype. It's faster.'" [6]

The research backs Lucas' admission. In fact, some studies report that weight-based bias is even stronger than biases related to race or gender. Researchers at Wayne State University in Detroit analyzed data from 30 years of studies and came to this conclusion: "People who are overweight are viewed more negatively in the workplace than those who are of average weight." [7]

Regardless of their actual competence, overweight employees are typically subject to coworkers' unfavorable stereotypes based solely on size. Those negative stereotypes include, "laziness, sloppiness, untidiness, lack of self discipline and control. Overweight people are also labeled as being unhealthy, often smelly and lacking in motivation, which can affect any employer's decisions." What's more, bias against weighted workers actually prevents people from even being considered for careers that require mobility or face-to-face customer contact. [8]

Yes BillyBob, though they would never say it to your face, your employer is actually embarrassed by your weight, and will try to hide you from customers because of it.

Is that fair, or even acceptable? Well, no. But it's still the world in which you live, and the simple fact is that taking charge of your health and your weight will not only help you feel better, it'll likely help your career as well.

Better Health—Inside and Out

That leads to the next benefit of eating with a lower-fat discipline: Better health, both at work and at home.

Physicians tell us that consuming less fat lowers the risk of heart disease, diabetes, and cancer. We often scowl at people who smoke or drink excessive amounts of alcohol, thinking, "She's giving herself cancer," or "He's drinking himself to the grave." Yet how often do we make those comments while we're scarfing down a double-decker hamburger and fries, failing to recognize that the fat we're eating does much of the same kinds of damage to our own bodies?

Back in 2003, the U.S. Surgeon General, Dr. Richard H. Carmona, sounded an alarm in his testimony before a Congressional subcommittee. Titling his remarks, "The Obesity Crisis in America," Dr. Carmona reported that "It's the fastest-growing cause of disease and death in America. And it's completely preventable." He went on to reveal that "nearly two out of three Americans are overweight or obese. One out of every eight deaths in America is caused by an illness directly related to overweight and obesity." Oh, and there's more.

"The facts are staggering," Dr. Carmona said:

> • In the year 2000, the total annual cost of obesity in the United States was $117 billion. While extra value meals may save us some change at the counter, they're costing us billions of dollars in health care and lost productivity. Physical inactivity and super-sized meals are leading to a nation of oversized people.
> • This year, more than 300,000 Americans will die from illnesses related to overweight and obesity.
> • Obesity contributes to the number-one cause of death in our nation, heart disease.
> • Excess weight has also led to an increase in the number of people suffering from Type 2 diabetes. There are at least 17 million Americans with diabetes, and another 16 million have pre-diabetes. Each year, diabetes costs America $132 billion. It can lead to eye diseases, cardiovascular problems, kidney failure, and early death. [9]

This is not top-secret information. We all know that being too heavy is harmful to our health, and so you'd think that our society would be steadily improving in the area, right? After all, we know that smoking can kill you. Voila! Over that past several decades, incidence of smoking has declined from 45 percent to about 20 percent. [10] But guess what? Apparently we're not listening when guys like the Surgeon General tell us the truth about how eating similarly harms our health.

In 1990, every state in the entire USA had an obesity rate of 15 percent or lower—that is, not more than 15 percent of its population was obese. [11] By 2011, not a single state in America had an obesity rate that low. In fact, 49 of our 50 states charted obesity rates higher than 20 percent, with only Colorado (at 19.8 percent) barely staying in the teens. What's more, according to USDA research, nearly two-thirds (32 of 50) of our American states have an "adult obesity prevalence rate" of more than 25 percent. In all, the USDA reports that one in three American adults nationwide (34 percent) is obese—a number that's more than double what it was in 1970. [12] In fact, over the last twenty years, not a single state has decreased its obesity rate; instead, in the last five years alone, eleven states have "overachieved" their way to an obesity rate of more than 30 percent of their residents. [13]

Fact is, according to a recent poll by the Gallup organization, roughly two out of three Americans (around 65 percent) admits to being overweight—but only one in four of us (25 percent) is trying to do anything about it. [14] Is it any wonder our fatter, flabbier nation is also seeing increases in incidences of weight-related illnesses?

When it comes to our health as it relates to our eating habits, we're often like the chubby lady who eats a Twinkie with a diet Coke, and then wonders why she's overweight. Or we gorge ourselves on chicken-fried steak with onion rings, then order low-fat frozen yogurt for dessert. It would be funny if it weren't so true.

But you don't have to be mixed up about your health anymore. You can enjoy healthful eating—and better physical experience as a result.

Now, I have to tell you, when I first heard the news that my health was in jeopardy, I was tempted to give up, to shrug and say, "Well, if I've got 10 years left, I'll just indulge myself and enjoy it." But that didn't last long, because I soon realized two things.

First, living out even 10 years in poor health just isn't an enjoyable life. It's a miserable one—and not the kind of life I dreamed of for myself. My only real choices were to live out 10 years in increasingly poorer—and thus limiting—health, or to live out a longer lifespan in increasingly better—and thus freer, more enjoyable—health. Looking at it that way, the choice was simple.

I had a second reason for choosing the better health a low-fat approach to eating provides, and it was something my doctor pointed out: My son, Tony. I realized that my health affects more than just me; it plays a huge part in the life of anyone and everyone who loves me. When it came down to brass tacks, it was my young son that captured my attention. Having grown up without a father myself, I was determined not to let Tony grow up without one. So I said to myself, "I'm going to do all I can to improve my health because Tony deserves to have a dad around as long as possible."

Guess what? Your family and friends also deserve the joy of having you in their lives.

By implementing a low-fat eating strategy, you'll improve your health and allow your loved ones innumerably more opportunities to share life with the irreplaceable you.

More Joy

Hey, if you weigh less, look better, find greater success at your workplace, feel better, and have more energy, you can't help but be happier. You've got more time and energy and motivation to experience the joy that life offers each day—to "seize the day" and actively pursue to the fullest that special life God gave you. Your "joy quotient" just got better, making your daily life experience something to look forward to instead of something to dread. Niiice.

These are just a few of the benefits that come from making one simple life change: Eating less fat each day. But too many men throw these benefits away because they think a Big Mac tastes better than a happy, healthy, joyful life. Fortunately, you don't have to be that stupid—and you can start enjoying a healthy lifestyle today.

Here's how…

Two:

First Steps

So, by now you're probably asking the obvious question:
How do I start?

Great question. You're smarter than you look. The next step is to figure out how much fat you actually need in a day. Not want, but need.

Living a full, healthy life full doesn't mean you deprive yourself of any foods or nutrients that your body needs. Many gimmick diets encourage you to load up on one kind of food and exclude others. Or there are diet programs that allow only a certain number of calories a day. Sure these approaches can help you lose weight, but most often they leave you feeling hungry and deprived.

Remember Rule #1?

A man should never be hungry.

Good news, bro! A lower-fat eating style offers plenty of food choices while allowing the necessary amount of fat our bodies require. You can eat when you're hungry, and eat until you're full.

Yeah, you're gonna love it.

How Much Fat is Too Much Fat?

Most Americans take in about 34 percent or more of their calories from fat. [15] Governmental and national organizations advise that it's okay for 25 percent to 30 percent of our calories each day to come from fat, and a number of diet systems rely on the 30 percent figure. [16] These diet systems also tell you just to eat smaller portions of the fatty foods you're already eating, and leave you feeling hungry as a result.

Recommendations aside, *your body only truly needs to take in between 4 and 6 percent of its calories from fat.* [17]

For instance, if you eat about 2400 calories a day (typical for an adult male), most government overlords will tell you that it's okay to eat up to 80 grams of fat each day. That, my friend, is a lot of blubber.

Truth is, all your body needs to be fully satisfied and functional is about 14 grams of fat a day (the equivalent of a single tablespoon of vegetable oil) [18] —or about 5 percent of your daily calories.

So how much should you have?

Well, it's a good idea to talk it over with your doctor before you begin any significant change of diet, but for the purposes of this book, I want you to feel confident that your *Dude, You Don't Have to be Fat* efforts are providing all the fat your body needs.

Let's agree that getting 10 percent of calories from fat will be an acceptable place to start.

Figuring Out Your Goal for Daily Fat Intake

To make it easy for you to figure how many fat grams you need to meet this goal, look at Weight Chart A on page 117. This will help you quickly determine what a healthy weight might be for you based on your height and body frame. Insurance companies use a chart like this (in fact, this chart is adapted from the standard one that Met Life has been using for decades—though it doesn't take every factor into consideration).

While this chart is not an infallible, rigid law, it will give you a general idea of what a healthy weight range for you might be. For example, let's pretend you're my friend, Jimmy-Gus, who is 6' 0" tall. With a large frame, you'd probably feel good weighing somewhere between 164 and 188 pounds. Not too tough.

Next, take your target weight and find the corresponding number on Weight Chart B (page 118). The fat grams recommended by Chart B allow for 10 percent of your daily calories to come from fat. That amount of fat intake each day will more than meet your nutritional needs. Back to Jimmy-Gus, then. If JG's target weight is 170 pounds, then he'd want to eat 28 grams of fat or less per day to achieve and maintain a lifestyle in that weight range.

What if you're not comfortable with having 10 percent of your daily calories come from fat? What if you want to eat in a way that delivers closer to 5 percent of your calories from fat? Or maybe you want to go up to 15 percent of your calories from fat? If something like that's the case for you, then here's a three-step, mathematical formula to help you figure out how many grams of fat you should have each day. Grab a calculator, and follow along—it's easy!

Step 1: First, you'll need to get an estimate of roughly how many daily calories it takes to maintain your target body weight. To do that, select your appropriate weight from Weight Chart A and multiply that number by 15. According to fitness guru, Tom Venuto, you need to consume about 15 calories per pound of body weight to maintain that weight,[19] so this will give you a quick, ballpark estimate of the maximum total calories that would be typical for each day. [20]

For example, let's say that Jimmy-Gus' brother, Johnny-Gus would like to weigh 180 pounds. He'd do the math this way:

180 × 15 = 2700 calories a day

Step 2: Next you'll want to find out how many of your total daily calories will be fat calories. So you'll multiply your "calories a day" by your goal percentage of daily fat intake. For instance, Johnny-Gus wants to cut his fat intake to 12 percent of his total calories, so he'll multiply his "calories a day" by 0.12, like this:

2700 × 0.12 = 324 calories from fat each day

Step 3: Finally, you'll want to translate your "calories from fat each day" into grams of weight (which is how fat is measured and reported on food nutrition labels). Since 1 gram of fat holds 9 calories, then your final step is to divide your "calories from fat each day" by 9 and round off the result. That yields a number which is your maximum daily allowance of fat grams. So, for Johnny-Gus, the math would look like this:

324 ÷ 9 = 36 grams of fat a day

This formula is not too tricky, and can help you set intermittent goals if you'd like to move gradually as you lower daily fat-eating. Be aware, though, that Step 1 in this formula doesn't account for your activity level. If you tend to be less than moderately active (for instance, if you don't exercise regularly or if you work at a sedentary job), you'll probably want to adjust Step 1 and use a multiplier of 13 or 14 calories per pound instead of multiplying by 15 calories per pound of weight.

"Spending" Fat

No matter what your goal, though, think of the daily grams of fat you've targeted as the amount you have to "spend" for the day. This gives you more freedom in making choices. If you have 37 grams to spend in a day, you can choose to spend them on a small amount of fatty foods, or you can spend them on an abundant amount of healthful foods. The choice is yours.

This leads us to more good news: Eating less fat actually allows you to eat more food! This was convincingly demonstrated during a study of men and weight conducted at Stanford University some years ago. Researchers discovered that overweight men and thin men actually consumed about the same number of calories each day—but the overweight men ate more fatty foods in their diets, while the thin men ate more in the way of complex carbohydrates and less in the way of fatty foods. [21]

I know it doesn't seem to add up at first, but it's true because fat has more calories than proteins and carbohydrates. My wife saw this principle in action once when she was having dinner with her father, a retiree in his 70s. Amy's dad was learning about how to lower his fatty intake each day, and she was helping him figure out how much fat he was eating in that meal. He was having a veggie "burger" along with a spicy side dish of Spanish rice and black beans.

"You've got about five grams of fat there, Dad," she explained.

He was amazed as his plate was packed with food. Then Amy went over to the counter and picked up two Oreo cookies.

"Two of these cookies have seven grams of fat," she told him. "So you can eat that whole plate of food for dinner, or these two cookies. Which would you want, and which would leave you wanting more?"

It wasn't a matter of counting calories. Instead, by focusing on grams of fat, Amy's father could eat his fill, get plenty of nutrients his body needed, and never feel hungry. All while losing weight.

How Much Fat Am I Eating Now?

Now that you know how much fat you need, it's time to find out how much you're already eating. This takes a little practice and discipline, but it's not hard. It really comes down to reading Nutrition Facts labels and writing down how many grams of fat you eat in a day.

By law, all prepackaged foods must include information as to how much fat is in each serving. For example, a box of apple and cinnamon flavored oatmeal in my kitchen tells me that one serving has 1.5 grams of fat. A serving in this case is one pouch of oatmeal. I usually eat two pouches at a time, so that means I'm getting 3 grams of fat for breakfast

(1.5 grams per pouch x 2 pouches). Not too tricky. A can of soup says it has 3 grams of fat per serving. In this case a serving is 1 cup, which means there are about two servings (or 6 grams of fat) in the whole can.

For more information about reading Nutrition Facts label, check out the How to Read a "Nutrition Facts" Label" chart on page 120 of this book. The fat content for foods that are not labeled can be found through Internet sites and books available at your local library or bookstore. Additionally, fat counts for fast-food and restaurant food can be found at the restaurant's Website or online in places such as fatsecret.com and calorieking.com.

For now, though, just check the fat content of what you're eating as you eat it. Pick up a small notepad or set up a memo file in your smart phone and, each time you eat, jot down how many grams of fat you've gobbled down. Include meals (breakfast, lunch, dinner) and any snacks in between (pay special attention to foods you eat while watching TV, as those are easy to forget). Do this kind of "fat accounting" for a week, and by then you'll know where you're getting your fat, and how much you typically consume in a day.

Formulating a Plan—and Recruiting a Friend

Once you've determined how much fat you typically eat in a day, compare that to the amount of fat you actually need. Chances are good that the amount of fat you eat is quite a bit higher than the amount of fat you actually need. Now that you are armed with that knowledge, you can start deciding what to replace in your eating plan.

The first two weeks of a *Dude, You Don't Have to be Fat* lifestyle are the hardest, so ask your wife or girlfriend or a buddy or the entire men's ministry group at your church to help you stay accountable—especially during this transition time. Let's face it—fat can taste good! In fact, not long ago Frito-Lay actually added more fat to their "healthy" baked chips just to make them taste better. [22] But when you tell people about your commitment, they'll help you stick to your plan—and they might even join you. We'll talk more about this in chapter seven (page 45).

Be aware that it takes a couple weeks for your taste buds to adjust to the taste of less fat. But they will adjust! Give yourself time. After a few weeks of eating low-fat and no-fat foods, eating fatty foods will actually seem downright disgusting.

Your body will adjust pretty quickly to the benefits of consuming less fat too—and it won't appreciate fatty meals you try to force on it afterward. For instance, my wife went several months without eating high-fat red meat (such as fast-food burgers or restaurant-prepared steaks) then casually had a higher-fat, fast-food hamburger when out with a friend. She didn't even think about it, as she was still within her fat target for the day ... until about three hours later when she was physically sick as a result of trying to cram a huge wad of fat into her now-clean and healthy system. Her body was telling her it didn't want—or need— that fatty junk!

Ready…Go!

In Part 2 we'll dig more deeply into your full *Dude, You Don't Have to be Fat* game plan and mindset, but for now do these two things to get started on your better life:

1) Determine how much fat you need each day.
2) Get out a sheet of paper and start writing down how much fat you're actually eating each day.

Dude, You Don't Have to be Fat

Do this for at least one week.

After a week of tracking your fat intake, it'll be time to start choosing foods that'll help you meet your new daily goal for fat consumption. That's where the fun begins—and the chapters in Part 3 will really come in handy.

But for now, tell a friend what you're starting, and let's get busy!

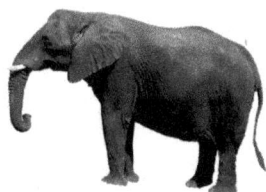

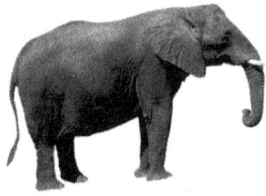

Part 2

Your Game Plan

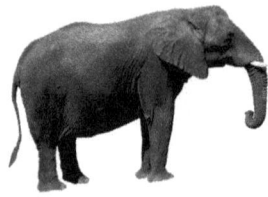

Three:
Fight S.M.A.R.T.

Muhammad Ali was getting his ass whupped.

It was 4:00 a.m. local time, October 30, 1974. Despite the ungodly hour, 60,000 people had still crowded into the boxing arena in Zaire to witness firsthand what had become known as "The Rumble in the Jungle." Muhammad Ali was, surprisingly, the underdog in this fight—a former champion trying to regain his claim to glory. The behemoth that stood in his way:

George Foreman.

Foreman, unsurprisingly, was the odds-on favorite for several reasons. He was the current heavyweight champion of the world. He was younger than Ali. He was stronger. He was a dominating boxer who had already knocked out 37 opponents. And perhaps most telling, he'd recently dismantled then-heavyweight champion Joe Frazier by knocking him near-senseless—and to the ground—six times in one bout.

Yep, Foreman had overpowered Smokin' Joe Frazier—the same guy who'd punished Ali with his first devastating defeat three years earlier. The outcome of this new fight was obvious, wasn't it? Most experts said Ali would need a miracle to beat big George.

Of course, most experts were wrong.

Before the Rumble in the Jungle, Muhammad Ali had spent months training and working out his strategy: "We're gonna dance!" he told his trainers. That was the game plan. Simply stay out of the way of Foreman's punching power, stretch the fight and let Ali's speed be the difference.

Then round one happened, and to even a casual observer, one thing was clear: Muhammad Ali was getting beat up all over the ring. In that first round, Ali quickly discovered that his original game plan was going to be woefully inadequate for this fight. And, while getting his lights punched out, he noticed three things:

1) The younger fighter was too fast—Ali couldn't dance quickly enough to stay out of his punching range.

2) George Foreman was a heavy hitter, but after taking a few hits Ali felt certain he could take Foreman's best punches, and then some.

3) Foreman was fighting for a knockout—he wasn't holding enough in reserve to last a full 15 rounds.

The rest, as they say is history.

Right there, between round one and round two, Muhammad Ali changed his game plan. No more dancing; he would employ instead a "rope-a-dope" strategy, back against the ropes, arms up to block the brunt of the hits, letting George Foreman wail away with punch after punch, counting on the younger fighter to recklessly tire himself out in the process.

Ali's trainers thought he was crazy. Everyone watching thought he was crazy. Any moment, it seemed, the fight would end with Ali tumbling unconscious to the mat. But every time Foreman finished a new flurry of blows, Ali would just grin at the heavyweight champion and say, "Hit me harder!"

By the eighth round, George Foreman was exhausted, punching wildly, barely able to control himself. So Muhammad Ali made history, finally stepping away from the ropes and suddenly taking the fight directly to the fading champ. The bout was over before round nine could begin. Muhammad Ali's new game plan had worked a miracle, knocking out the supposedly unbeatable Foreman to win back the heavyweight championship of the world. [23]

Your New Game Plan

If you're as bright as I think you are, then you know why I told you this story of Ali's historic triumph at the Rumble in the Jungle. Fast forward to today, and this time you get to play the part of Muhammad Ali. The role of George Foreman, that intimidating power puncher, is being played by Fat.

And let's face it: up to this point Fat has been whupping on you like a bully beats up a nerd in gradeschool.

Maybe you thought you were young enough to dance away from danger, that you could outsmart Fat using the same game plan you used back when you were young and reckless and on the top of the world. But here's the truth: Fat is winning. It's pounding your body, sapping your will, straining your relationships, hurting your self-esteem, and even wearing down your appreciation for this precious, short life God has given you.

Fat is planning to knock you out cold—and it will succeed unless you make a change.

It's time for a new game plan in your life, one that ends the rope-a-dope and lets you take control of this fight. One that lets you deliver the knockout punch instead of taking the hits. One that brings you the thrill of victory instead of the agony of defeat.

So here's what you're gonna do...

Fight SMART

That's they key to your *Dude, You Don't Have to be Fat* game plan, and it looks like this:

Mindset Change = Action Set Success

That means you begin pursuing your goals with a mindset change that naturally creates an action set for victory.

For Muhammad Ali, this formula that meant ditching an "avoid him" mindset for an "outlast him" strategy. That, in turn, created a whole new action set—instead of dancing and weaving, Ali adopted a defensive stance, using the support of the ring ropes to preserve his energy while protecting himself with raised arms and compacted posture. Next he attacked the mental toughness of his opponent, needling him with verbal taunts. Finally, he exhibited great patience, waiting for the bigger man to wear himself down.

Dude, You Don't Have to be Fat

Then—Boom!—the fight was over. His change in mindset had delivered an action set that brought home the victory.

For you, making a change in mindset means it's time for you to get off the ropes, to claim your "fridge benefits" by fighting SMART:

Simplify eating decisions.
  Make it easy to eat well.
    Act out love.
      Recruit allies.
        Take charge of your attitude

Let's learn more about what that means.

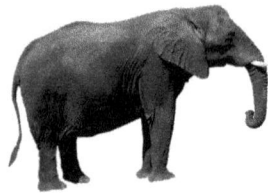

Four:
Simplify Eating Decisions

*The first step in your mindset change is to
simplify the rules of the fight.*

Here is where *Dude, You Don't Have to be Fat* excels because, unlike many other eating plans or "diets," there's only one thing that matters for your food health: Fat consumption.

Yes, other things such as sugar dosage and exercise and calorie counts can be important, but guess what? You don't have to worry about that tedious garbage. All you have to worry about is whether or not junk (i.e. fat fat fatty fatterson fat) enters your mouth.

That means anytime you're about to take a bite of something new, you just have to ask yourself one question: *How much fat is in this?*

The way you answer that question makes your eating decision a simple one. The principle looks like this:

Low-Fat or No-Fat = Good Eats.
NOT Low-Fat or No-Fat = Crap.

Remember back in chapter one when we figured out how much fat (in grams) you thought would be right for you each day? Make that number your target for maximum fat intake in a day, and then measure everything you eat against how much fat it forces you to eat—making sure you never eat more fat in a day than you've targeted.

Again, if that sandwich or cake slice or fruit salad (or whatever) comes in as a low-fat or no-fat intake, that's good eatin'. But if that sandwich or cake slice or fruit-salad-with-whipped-cream-and-tater-tots charts higher fat content, then that's junk your body doesn't want or need.

Wait...Don't I Need Fat?

"Mike," you say, "really, how intolerant are you? Everybody needs some fat in their food, so why all the hating? Can't we all just get along with fat?"

Well, no.

Here's the deal with fat in your diet. A small to moderate amount of fat is actually a good thing. It helps you to absorb vitamins A, D, E, and K, which in turn help strengthen your vision, skeletal system, and vascular health. It also helps regulate body temperature and provides protective covering for body organs and nerves. [24] Plus it adds flavor to food, which is always nice, right?

The problem is that we Americans don't eat small to moderate amounts of fat. Fact is, each day the average American (this means you) eats eight times more fat than the body needs. [25]

Nutritionists report that your body needs only "the equivalent of one tablespoon of vegetable oil" (about 14 grams of fat total) each day to function at optimal capacity. [26] Because fat is present, in varying levels, in such a wide variety of food, it's practically impossible for you not to get that small amount of fat required in your daily foodstuffs. Realistically, you'd have to be on a strict vegan diet or on some kind of semi-starvation eating plan in order to avoid getting that tablespoon of fat in your mouth on a normal day.

Trouble is, if you're like most people, you've managed to translate "one tablespoon of vegetable oil" to mean "I need to cram an entire stick of butter (about 91 grams of fat) into my mouth every day." [27]

Brain up, Dude. You don't need to push that much fat past your teeth today, or tomorrow or ever—let alone every day. In fact, I dare you to try eating a stick of butter every day for a week, just to see what it feels like. (Pretend it's some kind of disgusting Popsicle or something.) Now imagine eating that stick of butter 365 days in a row...or for two years...for ten years...for thirty years. No wonder you feel like Big Ol' Lard Man. When you abandon the natural plan for your body health and eat constant overdoses of crap, you feel like crap (and you start to look like it too).

Fat is Fattening (Duh!)

So the first thing you must understand that fat is fattening.

I know, that sounds like a "duh" statement, but you'd be surprised by how many guys either don't know or just refuse to believe that simple truth.

Fat contains more than double the amount of calories that an equal portion of protein or carbohydrates holds. One gram of fat contains 9 calories. One gram of protein contains only 4 calories, which is the same as one gram of carbohydrates. This is a problem because we know that calorie-dense foods are fattening, so a serving of something like fatty red meat will actually pack more weight on you on than an equal-sized serving of foods with low calorie density (such as chicken breast or extra-lean beef). As one nutritionist explains it, that means that "ounce for ounce, fat really is fatter." [28]

Additionally, fatty foods take longer to communicate to your brain that you are full. Health and weight loss expert, Dr. Louis Aronne, says that's because "fatty foods do not suppress the hunger hormone ghrelin as quickly or as much as protein does...and may not suppress hunger at all." This finding was confirmed in a study at the University of Leeds which monitored the hunger patterns of people who ate additional fat or carbohydrates at the start of a day. The carbohydrate eaters instinctively ate less food the rest of the day to compensate for the extra morning consumption. The fat eaters continued to chow down all day long like nothing had changed. [29]

This fatty fact of life showed up again in a unique study conducted by researchers at the University of California, Irvine. They examined how eating fatty foods (such as French fries and potato chips) influenced endocannabinoids in the body. Endocannabinoids are "natural marijuana-like chemicals" that "stimulate a biological mechanism that encourages gluttonous behavior." Their findings? When you eat fatty foods, it sends a signal to your brain "and then through a nerve bundle to the intestines. This signal then triggers the production of endocannabinoids" which, in turn, gives you a drug-like craving for more fatty foods. It's actually very similar to what happens to marijuana smokers when they get "the munchies" to go along with their high. [30]

What that means is, even after eating a lot fat, you can still feel hungry—which causes you to eat even more fat and which over time will engorge your body with fat.

Fat and Your Testicles

There's more. Not only does higher fat intake translate into body fat, it's actually dangerous for your manhood.

That get your attention?

According to a study by the journal of Modern Medicine, a high-fat diet tampers with your testosterone levels. Subjects in the study experienced a drop in testosterone levels of up to 30 percent simply as a result of eating one high-fat meal each day. Why is that a big deal? Well, the testosterone hormone in your body builds muscle, burns fat, boosts energy, strengthens your bones, combats depression, and raises your level of optimistic thinking. Oh yeah, and it also powers your sex drive. [31]

A high-fat diet also weakens other aspects of your masculinity. Consider: Doctors from Harvard University and the University of Murcia, Spain, studied hundreds of young men (ages 18-22) deemed to be in "optimum health" to gauge how their eating habits affected their ability to sire children. Their finding? "Junk food damages sperm thanks to its high fat content." [32]

Yep, guys who ate "high-fat foods such as biscuits, cakes, chocolate, crisps, takeaways and fried and processed foods" actually weakened their own sexual reproductive ability with their lazy eating habits. "Even if they [high-fat, fast-food-eating men] were a healthy weight and regularly exercised, their sperm was found to be less likely to survive the journey to fertilise an egg." [33]

Additionally, if you are indeed a fan of sex and your own testicles, there's even another reason you'll want to be careful about how much fat you eat. Prostate cancer ranks #2 in the list of most common cancers afflicting American men—and scientific studies have shown repeatedly that this kind of testicular cancer is linked to a man's dietary fat intake. In fact, Dr. Robert Cooper reports that:

> Researchers have known for a long time that prostate cancer is much less common in countries where the traditional diet is low in unsaturated fat … They also know that when men from Poland or Japan, where saturated fat intake is low and prostate cancer is rare, move to North America, their risk increases dramatically. The culprit, experts believe, is our all-American, extra-cheese-please, high-fat diet. [34]

So be good to your privates, men. Determine to simplify your eating decisions by evaluating any food according to only one criteria: How much fat's in there?

Remember:

Low-Fat or No-Fat = Good Eats.
NOT Low-Fat or No-Fat = Crap.

It really is that simple.

Action Set

Here are a few specific actions you can take to implement your new mindset to simplify eating decisions:

Keep track of how much fat you eat each day. (I might have mentioned this one before!) No matter what, don't eat more than the maximum amount you've determined is best for you and your goals. For me, that means I stay at about 29 grams of fat total each day. It usually breaks down as follows: About 5 grams of fat at breakfast; 6-7 grams of fat at lunch; 7-8 grams of fat at dinner; and a few snacks during that day that range from zero grams to 3 grams each. Figure out how that breaks down for you, and stick to it by keeping track of how much fat you eat each day. After awhile, you'll get into a good eating habit and it won't be as important to track everything every day ... but until you get there, make sure to write things down so you stay within your daily fat intake target.

Start reading the Nutrition Facts labels. Every packaged food you buy (including meats and cheeses) is required by law to list nutritional information. Near the back of this book (on page 120) is a diagram to help you understand what all those little numbers mean, but really, for the *Dude, You Don't Have to be Fat* lifestyle, all you need to know is what the "Total Fat" per serving is, and how many servings you expect to eat. This information is right at the top of the label, so look at it. You may be surprised.

One note: Some manufacturers try to make foods seem healthier by tinkering with serving sizes—so beware of that. Those companies think you're too stupid to understand that a teeny serving size is not realistic, even if it makes it seem like their food has less fat. So first ask yourself how many 'servings' of the food you would realistically eat, then multiply that by the total fat per serving to get your real fat amount.

Fill your life with fruit. Fruit is almost always the simplest, best choice for eating. With very few exceptions, just about every type of fruit is either fat-free or contains only trace amounts of fat. Plus, fruit is naturally sweet so it actually tastes good. (Hey, there's a reason why so many candies and desserts are fruit-flavored.) And fruit is abundant in our society—you'll find it in airports, at fast-food restaurants, in convenience stores, grocery stores, on street corners, and pretty much everywhere.

We'll talk more about this amazing group of food in chapter thirteen, but until then take this message to heart:

When in doubt, fruit it out.

Five:
Make It Easy to Eat Well

The second step in your SMART mindset change is to make it easy to eat when you're hungry.

Remember the cardinal rule of a *Dude, You Don't Have to be Fat* lifestyle? A man should never be hungry. That's not just empty talk—that's the real deal.

Food is awesome, and we should enjoy and be grateful for it. So when I'm hungry, I eat. And I keep eating until I'm not hungry anymore. The difference between me and you, right now at least, is that I make it easier to eat those things which are low-fat or no-fat than it is to eat the high-fat, junk foods that abound in our society.

But listen, bro, when you're hungry, you've got to eat.

Some people smirk disdainfully at that idea. They think like one college student in Louis Aronne's class did:

"Dr. Aronne," he said during a lecture on health and appetite, "I understand what you're saying about physiology, but isn't this really about laziness and lack of discipline? Weight loss is really simple. Just push away from the table."

So Aronne issued this challenge: "If you think it's so easy to push away from the table, I want you to try it. Don't eat until tomorrow's class."

The student took the challenge, confident he could easily go 24 hours without eating.

That lasted until about 3:00 in the morning, when he was so hungry he actually got out of bed to raid the refrigerator. His roommates laughingly reported the lapse the next day at class.

"Why did you eat?" Dr. Aronne asked.

"I didn't feel right. I was so hungry I couldn't sleep."

"Food has a physiological effect," Dr. Aronne explained to the rest of the class. "When overweight people eat less, they often feel just as he described ... as soon as they cut back on their calories or portions, they feel lousy and can't function." [35]

So let's face the fact:

When we're hungry, we need to eat.

Except in the case of occasional religious observances, denying a man's natural hunger impulse through fasting or portion control or premature meal cessation just doesn't do you any good.

I think fitness expert, Jackie Warner explains it best:

"Deprivation does not work! Nutrient deprivation is responsible for much of your weight gain. When you skip meals, your body thinks it's being starved, so it slows your metabolism and stores fat it would normally burn." [36]

So What Do I Do When I'm Hungry?

The point here, then, is you're going to get hungry, and you've got to eat. So what do you do when that happens?

Your society has stacked the deck against you in this regard. You can get high-fat junk on any street corner and in just about every corporate break room in the nation. In fact, it's easier to buy food that'll kill you than it is to buy a gun or a bottle of diet pills. So that means you have to take control of the situation and adopt the mindset that says:

I will make it EASY for me to eat well.

Remember Rule #3 of the *Dude, You Don't Have to be Fat* lifestyle? Eat great, lose weight, live well. That happens when you take control of your eating habits so they conform to the natural plan for your body. To do that you must train yourself to insist on creating a life that provides safe places for you to eat, to take charge of your surroundings. To take personal responsibility for the food that's available for you to eat when you're hungry.

Some gutless, lazy guys think they're powerless in this area, that all they can do is eat what other people provide for them. "That's all that was in the break room!" Flubbery Joe whines. "My wife put the M&Ms in the cabinet!" says Butterbean Billy. Whiners like these guys are just looking for an excuse to be fat and unhealthy. They want to blame someone else for their disappointing, unfulfilled lives. You're not that guy.

Truth is, you're not at the mercy of your surroundings, of your society, or even of your workplace. You control your own destiny—and your victory.

Think about your favorite football team. You know, for four hours each Sunday that team plays at its highest level, determined to score points and prevent the other team from scoring. Now do you think those guys win by ignoring football Monday through Saturday? Do you think they sit back and hope that somebody will have a play to run on first and goal? That they wait around until kickoff to see which team will oppose them? Of course not. Those guys spend all week planning and working and preparing so that, come Sunday, it looks easy to toss that quick out and then race up field for the touchdown. They work hard to manipulate their circumstances to optimize their chances victory.

Here's an idea: *What if you did the same thing?*

What if you actually were proactive instead of reactive about your hunger? What if you set yourself up so that, anytime you got hungry during the week, it was easy for you to eat well?

That's the crux of this mindset change. You've already simplified your eating decisions (low-fat or no-fat = good!), now all you have to do is make it easy to follow your own simple desires regarding food health.

Ah, such power you hold! So why aren't you using it?

Action Set

Here are a few specific actions you can take to make it easy to eat well:

Conquer your kitchen. This is where you take advantage of the second rule of this book: Food is not your enemy. Let's face it, you eat what's in your kitchen—so in order to make it easy to eat well you'll begin by stocking your kitchen with satisfying, low-fat and no-fat treats. I want to spend more time on this subject, so we'll discuss it in depth in Part 3 of this book. For now, just understand that your kitchen is going to make a big difference in your food health habits—and that's something you can get excited about.

Plan ahead. If you're like most people, tomorrow afternoon around 2:30 p.m. or 3:00 p.m., you're going to get hungry. What will you eat when that happens? If you work in an office building, chances are you'll wander over to the break room and pull a fat-capsule (i.e. candy bar or bag of chips) out of a vending machine. If you work outdoors, you'll likely grab a fat-heavy snack at a convenience store or nearby fast-food place. Basically, you're going to eat whatever is nearby, fat or no fat. After all, you're hungry.

Listen, no matter where you are, you shouldn't leave that snack choice up to chance. If you know when you'll likely be hungry, you can plan ahead and have something ready to stuff in your face at a moment's notice. And if you take charge of what that snack will be ahead of time, you can make sure it's something that fits your *Dude, You Don't Have to be Fat* lifestyle—something you enjoy and which delivers a low-fat or no-fat impact.

Same goes for when you plan to eat out, or plan to take a road trip, or just go to the movies. Look, you know you're going to do those things, and you know you're going to need to eat while they happen. So take the time to plan ahead a bit so you can satisfy that hunger craving with food that works for you instead of against you.

Going out on a business lunch this week? Check the restaurant's menu online and choose your meal ahead of time. Heading to the movies with your favorite girl this weekend? Plan your movie snacks before you smell the fat-packed popcorn in the lobby. Know your stomach starts grumbling mid-morning every day? Throw some good stuff for snacking into your desk drawer or on the shelves in the break room fridge. Planning ahead like this makes it easy to eat well. When the hunger hits, you're already prepared to eat.

If it's not low-fat or no-fat, don't buy it. This is such a no-brainer, I'm almost embarrassed to say it here … but I've found that most guys don't use their brains much when it comes to eating. So, look Dude, don't buy fatty food you don't want to eat.

This is related to the way you fill your kitchen, but applies to your broader lifestyle as well. Why buy food that you don't need, don't want, and which can actually hurt your body? If you invest in something, you're going to use it. If you buy a motorcycle, you're gonna ride it even if your wife doesn't like it when you do. If you rent that porn movie, you're gonna watch it even if it violates your own personal beliefs. If you buy that junk food, you're gonna eat it whether you really want to or not. You've already invested in your own temptation, and you're going to make it pay off.

Having high-fat garbage around and readily available in your life just makes it harder for you to eat well. So here's a great idea: *Don't buy it.* It's easy to avoid eating junk food when that junk food is nowhere around. Don't invest in it, and then you won't be tempted by it when you're hungry and looking for something to chew on later.

Now, on to more important things…

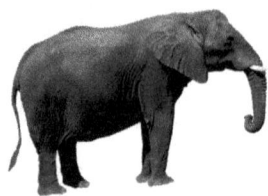

Six:
Act Out Love

The third step in your Dude, You Don't Have to be Fat *mindset change may seem a bit touchy-feely for some, but it's probably the most important mindset when you're fighting SMART.*

Why? Because this single thing is the core, basic, human motivation for why this book works: **Love.**

Whoa, partner! Don't roll your eyes at me and act like you don't need to hear this. Truth is, if you can't master this part of the *Dude, You Don't Have to be Fat* mindset, you will doom yourself to failure. Everything you do, everything this book is about, stems from this single mindset. So pay attention and get it right the first time, okay?

What I'm talking about here is agápē (pronounced "ah-GAH-pay"), a term ancient Greek thinkers and early Christian philosophers used to describe the purest, most selfless form of love.

Agápē is known as a love that's "not about what I can get, but what I can give." [37] It's defined as "a love generated by the will … *it acts for the benefit of the loved one* even when an act of love costs the lover everything" [38] (italics mine).

Listen to me now. The whole *Dude, You Don't Have to be Fat* concept is rooted in agápē, because for me (and for you, I think) that's what makes a healthy lifestyle worthwhile.

Remember, when I told you my story earlier in this book, how I faced a medical uncertainty that demanded a change in my eating and food habits? The thing that tipped me toward health and happiness was an energetic, joyful ten-year-old boy living in my household at that time.

"Your son deserves to have his father around for a long time," my doctor said to me—and he was right.

I love my son, I thought to myself. *Therefore, I will take care of his father. I'll do whatever it takes to make sure this child has a great father for as long as this life will allow.*

What's That Got To Do With Me?

Well, right here, right now, I'm challenging you to agápē the people you care about—and who care about you—by taking care of one of the most important people in their lives: You. And I'm telling you that in order for you to accomplish that, you've got to begin learning to agápē yourself with a selfless love that seeks your best benefit when it comes to the foods you stuff into your face.

No, that's not a contradiction. Your society tells you that loving yourself means indulging yourself, seeking to gratify your every desire regardless of how that impacts anyone else around you or the long-term consequences in your own life. And hey, that's a tempting way to live … for awhile. But the payback is awful, and you've already started to discover that for yourself.

When you learn to agápē yourself, you choose to act on your own behalf as if acting on behalf of a loved one—regardless of whether or not that love act satisfies a self-centered desire or feeds your ego or is convenient or strokes your inflamed sense of self-entitlement. In this context, often self-agápē is the least selfish thing you can do.

I love my son, therefore I will take care of his father. I love my wife, therefore I will work to be a strong, healthy partner for as much of her lifetime as I am privileged to share. I love my friends, therefore I will not hurt myself and subsequently hurt them with worry, disappointment, and loss.

You begin to understand what I'm talking about, yes? If not, take time to re-read the last few pages here until you do. Believe me, grasping this truth now will radicalize the way you live out the *Dude, You Don't Have to be Fat* lifestyle in the best, most lasting ways.

It's a Family Affair

Which leads me to the next point: When you act out agápē for yourself in terms of food health and pursuing lower-fat eating habits, by natural extension you are also acting out agápē for everyone in your family. Here's why:

You (and your spouse if you are parenting your children together) are the number one influence on your children's health—particularly in their eating habits that influence health. Dr. Robert Cooper reports, "Studies show that consciously or unconsciously, over-weight parents tend to teach their high-fat eating habits to their children. And that works both ways: If you provide nutritious, low-fat, high-fiber foods and set a positive example, you can influence your kids' eating habits for the better." [39]

Hey, check it out! You're a role model. Yay.

To some degree, your kids will live out whatever you act out. If you act out a lazy, careless, self-hurting lifestyle in the way you eat, don't be surprised when your kids do the same.

But what if you act out agápē toward your kids, if you model and lead them in a healthy, enriching lifestyle that enjoys good food without endorsing junk food? Well, trust me when I say it won't be long before you can literally see the difference in your children. So man up, bro. Be the agápē father your kids deserve.

FYI: Being a Fat Kid Stinks

If that's not enough for you, consider this: Being a fat kid stinks. Why would you want to give your kids that kind of childhood?

Here are the facts: [40] [41]

- In 1980, only about one in fifteen (less than 7 percent) of American children could be classified as "obese." A generation later, that number had risen to the point where about one of every five kids in America (19.6 per-cent) is obese. Don't believe it? Next time your visit your child's school, go ahead and count the number of heavy kids in the desks around the room.

• Fat kids grow up to be fat adults. One study of overweight 10- to 13-year-olds discovered that years later, when those kids were adults, almost all of them (about 80 percent) were still fat as grown men and women. What's worse, these fat kids who became fat adults tended "to have more severe adult obesity" than their peers who were thin as kids but fattened up as adults.

• Obese children are more likely to develop heart disease. In fact, more than 70 percent of these kids are at higher risk for heart problems than their non-overweight peers.

• Obese children are also high-risk for developing liver diseases, asthma, sleep apnea, type 2 diabetes, and early onset arthritis.

• Kids who are overweight also live life with higher emotional stress and lower self-esteem than their average-weight peers.

• Overweight children have diminished capacity to concentrate, and experience fatigue more easily, which in turn limits their ability for academic success.

• Heavy kids are more likely to experience depression and anxiety, as well as social discrimination that denigrates them and excludes them from peer groups.

• Several scientific studies that have followed fat children into adulthood reveal that these obese children grow up to be adults who earn less money and who are less likely to get married than their normal-weight peers.

• Guess what: The primary reason for the prevalence of childhood obesity in America is found in kids' high-fat eating habits.

Now think about this. You are the most influential person in regard to your child's eating habits. You are the role model your kids instinctively imitate. You have the power to create a lifetime of health and well-being for your children simply by being a person who will act out enough agápē for yourself and your loved ones to live out a lifestyle of healthy, joyful food experiences.

Get the message?

Action Set

Here are a few specific actions you can take to implement this new mindset in your life:

Love yourself—every day. You are a unique, important, valued person. Live each day that way! Wake up in the morning grateful for the opportunity to breathe again, to love again, to experience love again. Then let every food decision you make from that point on reflect that love, as if following an "If...then..." logical equation.

For instance, "If I love myself today, then I will pack my body with power food, not with fatty, junk food." "If I love myself, then I'll skip this fat-bombed donut and wrap my lips around a blueberry bagel instead." "If I love myself, then I'll choose a low-fat, grilled chicken sandwich for lunch instead of a heart-attack triple burger with fries." "If I love myself, then I'll eat well today so that I can love myself more tomorrow!"

Love the people who love you—every day. No man is an island, as they say. Anything that impacts you has an impact on anyone who loves you. When you are physically weak or emotionally self-destructive, your loved ones feel that pain with you. And often, they experience it with unique intensity because they feel helpless to help you (especially if you won't help yourself).

Similarly, when you take charge of your health, when you lead by example, when you become a man that your wife doesn't have to worry about, you give your loved ones an emotional lift that strengthens and inspires them. When you are the guy who is happy, healthy, and consistent in bringing good things to life, you become someone your kids look up to and a person who makes everyone around him better. Plus, you just enjoy loving and being loved more and more each day! So act out agápē toward those you love by being a man who protects and strengthens what they think is valuable: You.

Smile—every day. Your life is already better than you think it is. And by adding an agápē perspective to your eating habits, it's going to get even better than you currently can imagine.

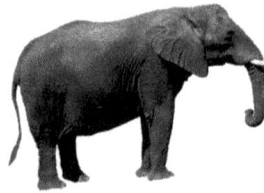

Seven:
Recruit Allies

The fourth step in your SMART mindset change is to recruit friends and family members to support your Dude, You Don't Have to be Fat *lifestyle.*

Ask any NFL quarterback what the key to his success is and you can bet it won't be long before he says two words: "Offensive linemen."

That's right, those nameless, Neanderthal, hulking hogs up front make all the difference between winning and losing, between a Hall of Fame career and becoming an afterthought in history's highlight reel. Every quarterback depends on those teammates for protection, support, and blind-side safety. A great quarterback will look average—and sometimes awful—standing behind a less-than-stellar offensive line. And an average quarterback can be great as long as his linemen give him time and protection.

I learned this in an unforgettable way in junior high, on my school's football team. I played defense—linebacker and occasionally defensive end. I loved it cuz all the coaches wanted me to do was "hit somebody, Nappa!" as hard as I could, play after play. Big fun.

During a scrimmage at one practice, those of us on defense were dominating our offensive teammates. I'd already blistered our running back a couple of times, and we'd all been harassing our quarterback into futility all day. On my side of the ball, we were having a blast. On the other side … not so much.

Finally our coach exploded in anger. He chewed out the offensive line with a few choice expletives (back then I guess it was okay to cuss out a 12-year-old). Then he told our quarterback to switch places with one of the linemen and instructed him not to block. He made the lineman the quarterback and ordered the ball to be snapped. I did what any blitzing linebacker would do: I blew past the non-blocking guy and dropped the new quarterback without mercy. My teammates piled on, leaving that guy grunting and sore. The coach pulled another lineman into the backfield, and now instructed others not to block. Those of us on defense could barely contain ourselves—we gleefully beat up every offensive lineman-turned-quarterback because no one was there to stop us.

Then the fun came to an abrupt halt. The coach sent our

regular quarterback into the backfield and returned the offensive lineman to their places. "Now," he said to them, "don't let these guys do to him," he pointed to the quarterback, "what they did to you."

Suddenly something clicked in the minds of those offensive linemen. They looked at me and my teammates with revenge in their eyes. The rest of the afternoon, they punished us, pounding the football down our throats, refusing to let us get close to the quarterback, until all we could do was watch them score touchdown after touchdown.

The lesson here, kids? If you're going to succeed, you need allies who are going to stand alongside you. You need "offensive linemen" in life who'll protect your blind side, shout encouragement, and sometimes kick you in the butt to get you moving in the right direction.

You need teammates who'll help you win.

What Difference Does It Make, Really?

Did you ever stop to consider why so many people trying to break addictions join groups? They need support! It's easy to make and break promises in our minds. But when we've made a commitment to someone else, actually said it out loud, maybe even written it down, it's a little harder to break our promise. Not impossible, of course, but definitely harder.

Support systems give us a place to feel safe and be honest about our needs, desires, and discouragements. These people can also help us feel loved when we don't feel very loveable, and our need to feel loved is important in breaking habits that have brought us comfort for many years.

Friends, family, church groups, and other support systems also can give you the encouragement you need to stick to your goals. This is simply an inherent part of human nature. Dr. Gavan Fitzsimons is a professor of marketing and psychology at Duke University. He explains this phenomenon by pointing out that humans are "social mimics," meaning that we tend to imitate the attitudes and actions of those in our social circles. Because of that, he says, "With more Americans overweight, scientists are [becoming] very interested in the subconscious cues that influence our eating habits." [42]

My wife tells a story of a time when she was traveling for business. She was eating dinner with a co-worker when the waiter brought out a tray of delicious-looking, fat-laden desserts. Amy was definitely tempted, but before she could say, "I'll take that chocolate mound thingy," her co-worker smiled at the waiter and said, "No thanks." Immediately it was easy for Amy to also say, "No thanks." She had an ally in her food-management goals, and in that situation, that made all the difference.

Research has shown that Amy's experience is not unusual—in fact, it's the norm. According to a recent Gallup poll of people trying to lose weight, more than two-thirds (68 percent) identify their "circle of friends" as an important source of help in reaching their goals. Additionally, according to a 2008 study by researchers at Harvard Medical School and the University of California-San Diego, "When one person slims down, those around him or her are more likely to lose ... If you have a close friend or a sibling who lives one mile or a thousand miles away, that person's weight loss or gain can have an impact on your weight." [43]

So guess what? If you surround yourself with people who support your healthy-eating goals, you'll increase immeasurably your chances of success—and you'll actually help them to eat healthier too.

But be warned, the opposite effect is also true. Researchers at Harvard recently studied a social network of more than 12,000 people. According to David R. Hamilton, PhD "They found that if one of your friends gained enough weight…it increased the chances of you also becoming obese by 57 percent." Dr. Hamilton concludes with this insight, "So just as we can catch a cold from a friend, it seems that we can also catch their habits. And, of course, we also spread our own. If we develop healthy habits, it might just be a blessing in disguise for our friends." [44]

Finding Allies for Healthy Eating

So as you can see, it's important for you to find people who will be consistent allies with you and who will cheer you on. The most obvious, and best, place to find that support is within your own family. Get your wife on board with your new lifestyle. (Honestly, she'll probably be thrilled because now it'll be easier for her to lose weight and eat well too.) When I changed to a low-fat eating style, my wife jumped right in with me—and we both benefitted from it. Even after more than 25 years of marriage, my wife weighed the same as she did when she was a college student on our wedding day. (I know, worked out great for me, huh?)

Also ask your kids not to fight you, or at least not to sabotage you, in regard to eating at home. When my son hit his teenage years, he was less than happy about the absence of abundant fatty snacks around the house. But he also knew how important it was for me to maintain food health in my daily life. So we reached a sort of tacit agreement. At home, he'd eat healthy stuff like the rest of us. Away from home, he'd eat whatever his teenage body could handle. For us, that worked out just fine—and it even helped Tony to pay attention to what we all were eating as well. I remember more than once he'd grab something at the grocery store, pause to read the Nutrition Facts label, and then toss it back on the shelf. "Way too much fat, Dad," he'd say to me with a grin. And we'd all move on. Awesome.

Of course, some families will just be against making changes in eating habits, and they're not likely to support you no matter what you do. That doesn't mean you can't make the changes, it just means they aren't going to be your cheering section. Find a couple friends who will join you instead. Or locate a support group in your church, or in your community through a health club, at your workplace, at a local hospital, or other organization. Share your goals for change with these people, and ask them to be the allies you need.

Support also comes from within. Not only do others support, cheer, and encourage you—you do this for yourself. For example, when you set realistic goals as to how much time it will take you to make the change to the *Dude, You Don't Have to be Fat* way of life, you're supporting yourself. When you read books like this one and learn tips and guidelines for making changes, you're supporting yourself. When you have a positive attitude about adding healthy food habits to your life, you're supporting yourself.

Take action today to find allies who will support you. Ask them to encourage you and hold you accountable to your goals. See if they'll join you in the change. And make sure you give yourself plenty of support through your own actions and attitudes. You deserve it.

Action Set

Here are a few specific actions you can take to implement your new mindset to recruit Dude, *You Don't Have to be Fat* allies:

Woo that Woman Again. When seeking out allies to support your *Dude, You Don't Have to be Fat* choices, you'll make no better teammate than your wife (if you are married), or your girlfriend, or whomever that special lady is in your life. When you two become a team, with shared values about healthy eating, you'll be nearly unstoppable. And honestly, your wife is probably more ready for this kind of change than you are—your lazy eating habits have definitely been holding her back. So here's your chance to make it up to her.

She can join you in this eating plan, or just help you make your home a place where your healthy food choices are easy and applauded—either way she wins. For starters, you'll look better, feel better, and be more fun to be around. But there's a bonus: Researchers recently studied 357 couples with at least one spouse who was overweight and trying to slim down. One year later, not only had the overweight person improved in weight and health—so did the spouse, even though the spouse was not participating in the weight loss program! [45]

Tell Your Friends Not to be Jerks. The overwhelming majority of your friends and relatives will support your decision to be healthier. After all, they love you and want you to be happy. However, polls do show that a minority of our "friends" may feel threatened by this kind of change, or even engage in a perverse kind of game where they try to get you to break, to join them in eating junk—just to see if they can do it.

Nanci Hellmich of USA Today reports that in a recent poll, "One-third of respondents (34 percent) have problems with how they've been treated by relatives and close friends during weight-loss attempts. They say their nearest and dearest have tried to lead them astray from their diets, teased them about their choice of foods or tried to short-circuit their plans." [46]

So, you know, you can cry about it and stuff your face with Twinkies. Or you can tell your friends not to be jerks who try to sabotage your attempts to improve your health and your life. You know what? Your real friends will happily get on board with that. And if you've got a work buddy or a church chum who can't get on board with that, then move on. You don't want to hang out with ignorant jerks who are actively trying to harm you—and you don't have to either. You can do better, bro. And you will.

Start a Dude, You Don't Have to be Fat *Club.* Chances are good that you aren't the only guy in your circle of friends who needs the lifestyle change described in this book. So go ahead and get a few of your buddies together and start a club that's all about getting healthier and happier in the way you eat. You can get together once a month or so for a low-fat party, watch the NBA games together, form a Facebook Group to post insights and updates, and more. This kind of shared experience will not only help you stick with your plan, it'll bring you and your friends closer and help build a lifelong bond between you.

Plus, you know, it's just fun to hang out with cool guys like you.

Eight:
Take Charge of Your Attitude

The fifth step in your Dude, You Don't Have to be Fat *mindset change is to stop whining and take charge of your daily experience.*

At the beginning, this may seem to be the hardest part of your food health transformation ... but just give it a few weeks and you'll discover it's actually the easiest thing to do. Of course, some of your friends won't see it that way. They'll shake their heads pityingly and speak condescendingly toward you while they scarf down a Double-Double with Cheese—and remain quizzically mystified that their blood pressure is through the roof.

Okay, this really happened, but I'm going to be deliberately vague about details, and I'm changing the name because I like the guy and don't want to embarrass him. A few years ago I was working at a local company and became friends with one of the executives there. Let's call him Freddy.

Freddy is a great guy—genuinely warm and friendly. Good sense of humor. Helpful. Smart. Football fan. Gets the job done, but also knows when it's time to stop working and enjoy life. Freddy is also about 100 pounds overweight.

So one day a bunch of us are sitting around the break room eating lunch and the conversation turns to food health. I explained (briefly) the *Dude, You Don't Have to be Fat* concept, and good ol' Freddy favors me with an expression of true pity. "So you can't eat the really good stuff like this," he says holding up his fat-caked fast-food lunch. "Man, that must stink. Too bad."

This guy actually felt sorry for me. He thought I was punishing myself by eating well! I tried to explain that I love the food I eat—it tastes great without threatening to kill me with fat overdoses every day. He simply couldn't believe me.

Then...

After we finished eating lunch, he said, "Just need to do one more thing before we head back to work." He mixed a laxative powder with water from the bottled water dispenser, and downed it all. "I'm on a diet," he said. "Need to lose a few pounds, so after I eat I take a laxative to help speed food through my system."

Now it was my turn to be mystified. Freddy's "health plan" was simply to eat garbage and then artificially incite diarrhea afterward. And he felt sorry for me? Puh-lease!

Fast forward to today, about three years later. The good Mr. Fred is still about 100 pounds overweight. I'm still at a healthy, enjoyable weight (between 175-180 every day), and I'm eating well—and loving it.

Perspective Matters

Here's why I tell you that story. Nobody likes being overweight, out of shape, and unhealthy. Everybody wants to be healthier and happier in daily life. Freddy and I wanted the same thing in that regard—but he thought eating and being healthy meant suffering and deprivation. I knew the truth: it means taking advantage of great-tasting food with lower-fat content, enjoying every bite—and the (diarrhea-free) life that comes after each meal.

Really, it's just a matter of perspective. When you think of living out *Dude, You Don't Have to be Fat*, do you see that as your punishment for years of unhealthy living? Or do you see it as your reward for choosing to act out agápē toward your loved ones and yourself?

Look at it this way. Let's say that as you're reading this book—poof!—a genie appears next to you.

"Master!" he says, "I'm here to grant your greatest automobile wish! Right here, right now, you can have any car in the world—money is no object. Fully loaded with all accessories. Anything and everything you could ever want in a car can be yours. Just make the wish and it's done. There's only one thing: This car has to last you the rest of your life. Once you own this beauty, there's no going back. You can never get another car from now until the day you die. Ready? Make your wish!"

Now, if you wish for and get, say, a brand new Bugatti Veyron sports car (about $2.2 million …diamond-studded instruments extra) [47] you've got a unique, valuable, exquisite marvel of mechanical engineering—and it's all yours. Way to go, Dude. I'm extremely jealous. Of course, now that you've got that mechanical masterpiece, what are you going to do with that car over the next 50 years?

My guess is that you're going to do your best keep that sweetheart in peak, pristine condition. You're going to take pride and joy in caring for that car. You'll probably pump high quality gasoline into that tank. You'll probably change the oil regularly, keep it washed and waxed, avoid getting into accidents, protect the interior from cigarette burns, park it carefully to avoid dings and dents, and generally show it off to friend and family member alike.

My guess is you'll never apologize to anybody for taking good care of that car.

Hey, it's got to last you a lifetime, right?

Better keep it in good shape so it'll perform the way you want it to day in and day out for the rest of your life. And your friends are never going to feel sorry for you about owning a near-priceless automobile. No one is going to say to you, "Wow, it's too bad you have to put gasoline in that Bugatti, when it'd be a lot cheaper and a lot easier just to fill your tank with mud." No sympathetic pal is going to shake his head and say, "Man, how your life must stink. I mean, you have to drive around in a beautiful, luxurious Veyron instead of just taking a beat-up skateboard everywhere you go. What a shame for you."

You see my point here, don't you? It's all about perspective. Some people will act like you're missing out on life by eating well and living well … but they're just morons with a warped view of life. Listen to me now:

God has given you an eternally unique, priceless, exquisite marvel of biological engineering—and it's all yours. There's only one thing: This fantastic body of yours has to last you the rest of your life. It's the only one you get, bro. And it's awesome … so why would you feel sorry for yourself about doing your best keep that hunk of awesomeness in beautiful, peak, pristine condition? Why should anybody?

Some guys act like it's weak or girly or embarrassing to take control of how they eat. That's just stupid. "Guys need to understand that food is fuel for your system," says Dr. Kim Bruno. "You wouldn't put bad fuel into your car, or into your boat. So why would you put bad fuel into your body?" [48]

So, yeah, some of your buddies may smirk and scoff and treat you with a little condescension. Forget them. They're filling their gas tanks with mud—and they're paying the price for it. They just don't want to admit it yet.

You've Got the Good Life

I always laugh when someone deigns to feel sorry for me and my *Dude, You Don't Have to be Fat* lifestyle. You know what I had for dinner tonight? A generous helping of tasty, home-style lasagna (see page 178), garden-fresh, seasoned green beans, cut-fresh honeydew melon, and a hunk of gooey chocolate lava cake (see page 198). I felt like I was eating at a fine restaurant—even though I was sitting in my own kitchen. Tomorrow for lunch I'll probably have shredded chicken barbecue (page 174), a super-fruit smoothie (page 215), and a sticky sweet cinnamon roll (page 209).

Does it sound like I'm suffering? Do you think I'm moping around, whining because I get to eat delicious, low-fat food that makes me feel good and doesn't harm my body in the process? Keep dreaming. I love it—and you can too.

So when the whiners and pitiers come around, or when you're tempted to feel like you're punishing yourself by choosing to eat and live well, remember to take charge of your attitude.

When your work buddy is choking down a fat-bomb of prime rib with a side order of death-fried onion rings, remind yourself that with your *Dude, You Don't Have to be Fat* approach to eating, you've got it all. You don't need that fatty junk to enjoy your life to the full. Your healthy, joyful life—and your peak-condition body—is better than that.

You may not believe that wholeheartedly just yet, and that's okay. But give it a few weeks and I guarantee you'll feel differently. Really, it's just a matter of perspective.

Action Set

Here are a few specific actions you can take to implement this new mindset:

Never Apologize for Eating Well. When your friends are chugging brats and sodas, don't act sheepish or apologetic for digging into an extra-lean burger with a bowl of strawberries-n-blueberries on the side. Who gives a rat's bum what those guys think about what you eat—and whether they want you to join them while they drown in fat? You do what tastes good—and is good—for your body, and make no apologies. There's joy in that freedom to eat well—so enjoy it and don't let your attitude be influenced by ignorant, lazy people who can't keep up with you.

Remember Duke Raynald III. In the mid-14th century, Raynald III was the son of Princess Eleanor and ruler of his father's lands in the Netherlands in Europe. He was also a big tub of lard, earning himself the nickname Crassus ("The Fat"). As often happened back then, Raynald feuded with his younger brother, Edward, who aspired to rule in Raynald's place. They went to war. Edward prevailed and captured his big brother. At that point, it would have been unseemly to execute the fat tub, so Edward did the next best thing. He had Raynald placed in a cell in the castle of Nieuwkerk (presumably by tearing down a wall and then rebuilding it).

The doors and windows of Raynald's jail were always open. "My brother is not a prisoner," Edward used to proclaim. "He may leave when he so wills." So why didn't he take his freedom? Because the guy was just too fat to fit through any opening.

To compound his troubles, the usurper Edward delivered abundant food to his brother's cell. Ol' Crassus could never say no to a tasty morsel, and so he spent the next decade behind bars, literally a prisoner of his own fat body. [49]

So next time you're tempted to feel sorry for yourself or to join your friends in feeling that it's a hardship or sacrifice to turn down a fat-laden food item, remember the life of Duke Raynald III. Let that be a catalyst for you to take charge of your attitude. Eating well is no punishment; it's the reward that'll set your skinny butt free.

Don't Punish Yourself with Rewards. This action item deserves a little extended attention, so let's talk about it for a minute.

Many diet plans make "rewards" a key element in their programs. They say things like, "Give yourself a treat and cheat every once in awhile. If you've worked hard to eat well all week long, you deserve a few less-than-healthy meals on the weekends." Or "Go ahead and buy yourself a new CD or jewelry to reward yourself for eating well."

What a bunch of horse excrement. Seriously, that's the most ignorant advice I've ever heard. Don't waste your time listening to it. First, it assumes that you're punishing yourself by eating well (which, clearly, you are NOT). Second, it just doesn't make sense. Imagine if we used that same kind of thinking in regard to a marriage, or a job.

"I've gone an entire week of having sex only with you," you say to your wife. "Therefore, this weekend I'm entitled to cheat on you with any drunk chick I can pick up during happy hour on Saturday night." How's that gonna fly in your home, Sailor?

Or what if you say to your boss, "Look, I've showed up for work for 40 hours this week. Therefore, you owe me a new watch or the latest James Bond 3D movie on Blu-ray. Well, I'm waaaiting!" Try that tactic with your boss two or three times, and then let me know how your new job hunt goes.

Idiotic, right? Regardless, many people assume that kind of self-sabotage is good thinking. They need to listen to people like nutritionist, Lisa Dorfman, who points out what should be obvious. "Special treats have a way of becoming everyday treats," she says sagely. "They're a relapse in the making. But if you make them inconvenient, you'll eat them less often." [50]

If that's not enough for you, then consider the science of behavior and motivation. In one study, dieters were placed into two groups. One group was promised a cash reward for reaching weight loss goals. The other was promised...well, weight loss and all the benefits that come with that. The ones receiving cash lost weight, then put it back on, yo-yoing and in some cases actually weighing more at the end of the study than they did at the beginning. Those without a reward system lost weight—and kept it off over time. Another, similar study 10 years later confirmed the same results with one significant difference: the folks in the reward group often just gave up and dropped out completely when they couldn't earn their rewards. [51]

So don't fall prey to the thinking of losers who've decided that eating junk is a reward for eating well. Change your attitude to reflect the truth that the reward of a *Dude, You Don't Have to be Fat* lifestyle is a lifestyle full of not being fat. Got it?

Good.

Part 3

Eating Well
at Home or Away

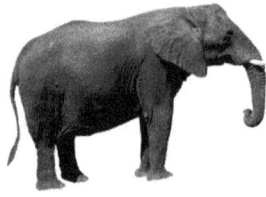

Nine:
Pantry Power

Okay, it's time for a pop quiz. Ready? Here goes.

1. How many American men are overweight?
2. How many American men don't prepare their own meals?

I'll give you a hint: both answers are the same.

Nearly two-thirds of us guys in America (64 percent) are overweight. Likewise, 64 percent of us don't prepare our own meals. [52] See a connection? I do. Guys are socially trained to be aggressive, take-charge people who lead everywhere ... except the kitchen. For some reason, we become passive, timid pansies as soon as we step into the shadow of the refrigerator.

Well, it's time for your manhood to assert itself; it's time to conquer your kitchen and take control of your eating life. I'm not saying you need to kick your wife out of the kitchen if she likes being there, but I am saying you need to have the courage to influence what happens behind your own pantry doors.

So far, you've learned some pretty important things. You've adopted the three rules of a *Dude, You Don't Have to be Fat* lifestyle:

1. A man should never be hungry.
2. Food is not your enemy
3. Eat great. Lose weight. Live well.

You've taken time to determine what your daily fat intake should be (see page 22). You've learned to think and fight SMART:

Simplify eating decisions.
Make it easy to eat well.
Act out love.
Recruit allies.
Take charge of your attitude

Now it's time to exert some Pantry Power in your home.

What do I mean by that? I mean it's time for you to take control of the food you stock in your pantry, in your cupboards, and yes, in your refrigerator. The goal here is simple:

Out with the bad
(high-fat, low-nutrient junk food)

In with the good
(low-fat and no-fat tasty treats that fill you up and nourish your body).
  Here's what we know:
• One-third of what the average guy eats, according to a University of California, Berkeley study, is "pure junk that provides no nutritive value." [53]
• If "pure junk" is in your pantry, you're probably going to eat it.
So you're going to be an above-average guy and stock your kitchen ONLY with good stuff that tastes great and gives you a body that you (and your wife or girlfriend) will be happy to have around. This starts, obviously, with what you buy at the grocery store, so in this section I'm going to walk you through the aisles and show you how to buy the good stuff, and how to avoid the bad.

First: The Food Groups

If you already know this part, feel free to skip to the next section. But if you're not sure about it, or if you just want a little refresher, read on. [54]

There are five basic types of food that we all eat:

Protein Foods. USDA describes these as meat, poultry, seafood, eggs, nuts, seeds, and processed soy products. (Some beans and peas also contain protein, but they're categorized as vegetables anyway.)

Dairy Products. This includes all milks, fortified soy beverages, yogurts, dairy desserts (like ice cream), and of course, cheese.

Grains. This refers to "whole" grains and "enriched" grains. Whole grains include foods which use whole grain as ingredients (such as whole-wheat bread, whole-grain cereal, whole-grain crackers, oatmeal, and brown rice). The disturbingly misnamed "enriched" grains include products that use refined (processed) grains as ingredients, such as white bread, enriched pasta, enriched-grain cereals and crackers, and white rice.

Fruits. All fresh, frozen, canned, and dried fruits. Also fruit juices (i.e., liquid fruit). For instance, this would include oranges, orange juice, bananas, apples, apple juice, grapes and berries, raisins (dried grapes and berries), melons, and so on.

Vegetables. This is the largest of the food groups, with several subcategories as follows:

• Dark-green vegetables. (All fresh, frozen, and canned dark-green leafy vegetables and broccoli, such as spinach, romaine, collard, turnip, mustard greens, and broccoli. This applies to both cooked and raw produce.)

• Red and orange vegetables. (All fresh, frozen, and canned red and orange vegetables, cooked or raw. This includes produce like tomatoes, red peppers, carrots, sweet potatoes, winter squash, and pumpkin.)

• Beans and peas. (All cooked and canned beans and peas, such as kidney beans, lentils, chickpeas, and pinto beans. Note: this subcategory does not include green beans or green peas.)

• Starchy vegetables (All fresh, frozen, and canned starchy vegetables such as white potatoes, corn, and green peas.)

• Other vegetables. (This catch-all subcategory refers to all the rest of the fresh, frozen, or canned vegetables, cooked or raw, such as green beans, onions, and iceberg lettuce.)

USDA MyPlate

With those food groups in mind, the USDA has created a recommended "plate" breakdown to help us morons out here to visualize the food we suck down each meal. You can see the graphic of this "MyPlate" on page 119 near the end of the book, but I want to tell you a little about it here. According to the MyPlate recommendations, your best meal is one where you do the following:

- Fill half your plate with fruits and vegetables.
- Keep protein servings at less than 25 percent of your place (typically about 5 ounces a day).
- For grains (such as breads, rolls, rice, cereals, and the like) shoot for about 25 percent to 30 percent of your plate. More importantly, make sure your grain-based foods include plenty of whole grains. USDA suggests a minimum of half the grains on your plate be whole grains.
- For dairy, USDA suggests about 1 cup per meal, which could be in a glass of milk, or in cheese in an entree, or in yogurt or any other dairy variation on your plate.

Now, I'll tell you right now that in my experience the some USDA dietary guidelines have not always delivered the results I desired, but I'll also say that this MyPlate breakdown looks pretty good from a *Dude, You Don't Have to be Fat* perspective. And now that we know what kinds of foods are out there, and in what kinds of proportions we want to eat those foods, we can hit the grocery store with a clear sense of purpose and confidence that we'll get exactly what we want—and what we need.

Before You Go...

One note here: Before you go to the store remember a few key things from your SMART mindset. First, you want to simplify your eating decisions after you bring your food home, so as you shop keep one question in mind: "How much fat is in this item?"

If it's low fat or no fat, that's good—go ahead and buy it. If it's not low fat or no fat, well, to quote the immortal Dionne Warwick, "Walk on byyyy!"

"No fat" is pretty easy to understand, but how do you know how much is actually "low fat"? After all, lots of foods describe themselves as "diet" "healthy!" or "lower fat!" that aren't actually low fat under the *Dude, You Don't Have to be Fat* thinking. For a definitive answer, first check what you identified as your maximum daily fat intake back in chapter two. Then allocate how much fat you want to "spend" during eat meal and snack of your typical day of eating, and buy accordingly.

For instance, I mentioned to you before that I stay at about 29 grams of fat total each day. I usually break that down as follows: About 5 grams of fat at breakfast; 6-7 grams of fat at lunch; 7-8 grams of fat at dinner; and a few snacks during that day that range from zero grams to 3 grams each. So when I'm buying food at the store, I use those allocations as a guideline for knowing whether or not something is "low fat."

If I'm planning to have a grocery item as a main dish for dinner, then I won't buy it unless it has 8 grams of fat or less per serving. (And often I'll insist on less than 8 grams in a entree, simply because I know I'll be eating side dishes or desserts with my main dish, and I'll want to "spend" a few fat grams on the side dish or dessert as well.) Likewise, if I'm buying a snack item or a dessert item, I typically won't buy anything that packs in more than 2-3 grams of fat per serving. For me, any snack higher than that would NOT be low fat. Make sense?

The second thing to remember before you go shopping is a one of the action sets in your make it easy to eat well mindset:

Plan ahead.

Never go to a grocery store without knowing what you're there to get. Sure, you'll probably end up with a few extra things in your cart—and that's okay. But 90 percent of what goes on the checkout counter should be items you actually planned, and wanted, to buy.

My wife and I will usually sit down for about 15 minutes before we go shopping and make a list of good stuff we want to come home with. First, since we typically eat dinners together, we talk about what we want to eat for dinner during the week (including what we want for leftovers). Then we list the low-fat ingredients needed for those meals. Next I think about what I'm going to want for breakfasts and lunches during the week, and I write down the supplies I need for those meals. Then I brainstorm a list of several tasty, filling snacks that I'll be happy to see whenever I get the munchies between meals.

Voila! When I plan ahead like this, I bring home enough food to last me all week long—and I make sure it's all good food that won't hurt my body. The results? Whenever I'm hungry, I always have "fridge benefits" waiting for me because anything and everything I could want is right within my reach.

No Crazy, Offbeat, Hard-to-Find Stuff Allowed

One other side note here: I hate books like this that tell you to buy crazy, obscure brands and products like "Uncle Fester's Fat-Free Baconella Cornpuppies" or something. For instance, I read a *New York Times* bestselling book recently where the author told me, with a straight face, to go out and buy "hemp sprouted bread, Tuno, chicken-style seitan, and organic sandwich crèmes."

Whaaa? I have no idea what that junk is, let alone where to buy it.

I'm guessing you're more like me than like that Tuno-loving writer. Guys like us? We shop at normal places and buy normal food that's on the shelves pretty much anywhere you go in these fine United States. So here's the promise I make to you now:

At the time of this writing, anything I tell you to buy at a grocery store, or any ingredient used in one of the recipes in the Mini-Cookbook for Men later in this book, could be found at a regular, national grocery store like Walmart, or Safeway, or a Kroger chain store (such as Kroger, Ralph's, King Soopers, City Market, Smith's, Fry's QFC, etc.).

Advertising Code Words

Now, one last thing before we go shopping.

The food industry knows that fat is an issue for many people and so they've created marketing code words to attract guys like us. They splash these codes in big print on their products, hoping we'll trust their advertising and buy their products without asking questions. Yes, it's actually helpful to have marketers point out lower-fat options in easy ways … but when was the last time you trusted an advertiser's claims, really? Better to know exactly what these people are talking about when they want us to buy low fat advertising.

To help us in that, the Food and Drug Administration has created guidelines for advertising descriptors in regard to low-fat foods. In order to use one of these descriptors lawfully, food producers must be able to prove their product meets the criteria described.

I've included a cheat sheet of those terms for you on the next page. Look it over, and feel free to photocopy this cheat sheet. Take it to the grocery store with you next time you shop—you'll find it to be very helpful.

All right, I think we're ready. Let's hit the aisles.

Cheat Sheet:
Advertising Code Words [55]

Code Word	What it Means	Advice
Fat-Free	Less than 0.5 (one-half) gram of fat per serving.	It is strange that something "Fat-Free" could actually contain up to one-half gram of fat … but that's not usually a big deal. Enjoy "Fat-Free" as much as you want.
Low-Fat	3 grams of fat (or less) per serving.	Like "fat-Free," this is a good target for you—enjoy!
Reduced-Fat	A minimum of 25 percent less fat, per serving, than the original version.	This really doesn't mean much for higher fat products, so beware this code word—it can be deceptive.
Light	Half the fat, per serving, of the original version.	This may or may not be significant, depending on the fat content of the original, so be sure to check the actual fat grams per serving first.
Lean	Less than 10 grams of fat per serving, including less than 4.5 grams of saturated fat, and less than 95 milligrams of cholesterol.	Not bad, but not great. Use this only if you can't get Extra-Lean.
Extra Lean	Less than 5 grams of fat per serving, and less than 95 milligrams of cholesterol	FYI—when it comes to meats, this is the good stuff. Get it if you can.

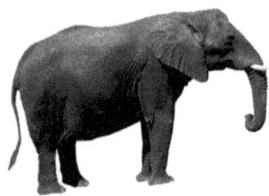

Ten:

Shopping for Proteins

When it comes to proteins, the things you'll be buying here include meats, poultry, eggs, fish, nuts, and seeds.

Now, many guys think that meat should be the main portion of a meal, with bread, fruits, and vegetables as the "side" dishes. I admit that I often think that way myself. Still, as you're shopping, keep in mind the MyPlate framework and stay open to the idea that your meat may actually be the "side" dish that fills only about a quarter of your plate instead of the center of it. This is particularly true in regard to red meat; poultry may be different however.

First Let's Talk about Red Meats

These are probably the meats you're most familiar with, and the term refers to meat that is typically dark red (bloody) before cooking. This includes beef (hamburgers, steaks, and such) as well as lamb and some wild game like venison, ostrich, elk, duck, buffalo and the like. This is probably my favorite category for a main dish, and I'm betting you're pretty fond of it too. It's also one of the top three sources of dietary fat for Americans. [56] And because it's used everywhere in everything, it can be deadly for otherwise smart guys like you and me.

Some folks (usually vegans or vegetarians, though some doctors as well) will tell you to cut red meats from your diet completely. Others (like Atkins dieters and beef industry advocates) will tell you that it's "what's for dinner," and you should eat as much as you can as often as you can. The truth lies somewhere between those two extremes.

So, we have to be smarter than our society when it comes to red meats. Fortunately, it's not too hard to do that.

Here's the rule on red meat: *Always insist on "extra lean."*

That means you'll be getting meat that has less than 5 grams of fat per serving (about 4 ounces of meat). That's plenty of meat for a meal, and it's actually a pretty good fat allocation for the main dish in a meal as well. Pretty simple, but it takes a proactive mindset when you're in the grocery store.

Check out the hamburger section next time you're at Walmart. Typically you'll see three or four kinds of ground beef there. The default is usually ground chuck (20 percent fat content—or 21 grams of fat for a quarter-pound burger) or ground round (15 percent fat content—about 17 grams of fat for a quarter-pounder). Stay away from that garbage. It tastes greasy and gross, and it's unnecessary to punish your body with that much fat just to enjoy a burger.

"Lean" packages of ground beef can seem appealing. These are the ones that sport that "93/7" notation on the front, meaning they contain 7 percent fat (and 93 percent meat). A four-ounce serving (that is, a quarter pound, pre-cooked) of this beef charts at about 8 grams of fat. Not bad if you're out to dinner with friends, but in your own home, it's still double what you need or want. Unless there are special circumstances, I'd say to skip this too.

Finally, you'll find exactly what you're looking for: That glorious package labeled "96/4" or "Extra Lean."

Now you're in business! A quarter-pound serving of this tasty burger-maker contains only 4.5 grams of fat. Bingo! You've hit the jackpot. Not only is this lean beef tastier and cleaner, it delivers a low-impact fat yield you can enjoy in everything from a casserole to a crock-pot supper to pizza topping to, of course, a juicy quarter-pounder with cheese and ketchup. So when buying ground beef, sort through the mess and pick up the gem: "Extra Lean 96/4" ground beef is all you need for the rest of your life.

It's a little harder to find Extra Lean steaks, but not impossible. If you're looking for something tasty, but low fat, to grill at your next tailgating party, I'd recommend extra lean, cube steaks from Walmart, seasoned with minced garlic and onion, and black pepper. Delicious—and only 1 gram of fat per ounce of meat (or 4 grams of fat per traditional serving size).

Be sure to check the weight on your package of steaks and then do the math to figure out how many ounces of fat are in your individual streaks. For instance, if your package holds one pound of meat, and there are three steaks in the package, then you'd figure: 16 ounces divided by 3 = 5.3 ounces per steak. That, in turn, yields 5.3 grams of fat per steak, which should be fine.

As a rule, cuts of beef that are marked "prime" (as in "prime rib") are NOT lean. Step away from the meat counter when you see that—you don't need it, and your body doesn't want it.

Meat marked "select" or "choice" are lean cuts and closer to what you're looking for ... but they still don't meet the "extra lean" standard. Occasionally, thin-sliced strip steaks (such as New York Strip Steak) can be acceptable for including in a meal—but be warned that strip steaks like this are rarely enough for a main dish. Go ahead and enjoy them as a side dish, but be sure you also fill the bulk of your plate with fruits and vegetables to fill your stomach.

Other red meats, such as lamb, buffalo, ostrich, and wild game are not as obvious as beef at your grocery store, but sometimes you can find them there. For instance, today at Walmart I found a nice selection of low-fat bison steaks—only about 3 grams of fat per 4 once serving. If you like bison, that's a good option anytime for you. Beware of ground bison though (i.e. "bison burgers"). Ground bison tends to come from fattier cuts and carries significantly more fat grams per ounce.

Ostrich steaks are also worth trying on the rare occasions when they show up on the shelves at your local store. This red meat is actually leaner than chicken, and has a beef-like flavor that's delicious, especially when it's seasoned well. I had it for the first time a few years ago when one of my publishers took me to an upscale restaurant to celebrate the release of a book. The waitress recommended it as a low-fat option, so I said, "Why not?" Turns out it was delicious. After that I found a wild game dealer locally who could special order ostrich steaks for me, so every now and again I'll treat myself to that. However, it only shows up seasonally in most regular grocery stores—and sometimes not at all. But if it does make an appearance on a Kroger or Walmart shelf near you, give it a try. I think you'll like it.

Regardless of what kind of meat or wild game you buy, make sure you still hold it all to the "Extra Lean" standard—don't buy any cut of meat unless it contains a fat load of about 5 grams or less per serving (about 4 ounces or one-quarter pound of meat). Just don't do it. You don't have to and—here's the surprise for most people—extra lean cuts actually are higher grades of beef. They taste better and are more filling … and did I mention they taste better?

Remember this when shopping for red meat: your best option is to always going to be to insist on "extra lean."

Chicken Chat (Poultry and Such)

When eating poultry, it's quite a bit easier to sort through the options. Basically it boils down to these two guidelines:

• Buy only "white meat"—that is, chicken breast or turkey breast. (Avoid dark meat like drumsticks, wings, and so on.)

• Always buy skinless poultry, or remove the skin yourself before eating. There's just too much fat in the skin.

White meat from chicken or turkey is one the best meats you can have in your diet. Dark meat? Not so much. Dark meat contains about 50 percent more saturated fat (plus it tastes kind of greasy and disgusting). Breast meat, though, is remarkably lean and tasty. A four-ounce serving of boneless, skinless chicken breast contains less than 3 grams of fat (2.66 grams to be exact). Likewise, a four-ounce serving of turkey breast yields less than 2 grams of fat (1.88 grams). That's excellent low fat, "extra lean" content for any meat.

Now, one thing to be aware of is that four ounces of white meat chicken or turkey is usually only about half of a breast cut of meat. That's actually about right for most of us, but sometimes I like to eat the whole durn breast, and I'm guessing you might feel the same way. That's fine. Because both chicken and turkey breast are so low in fat, you can eat a full breast cut (about eight ounces) and still only take in about 5 grams of fat for chicken and 4 grams in turkey.

Be aware though, that a surprisingly high amount of fat is present in poultry skin. For instance, one 8 ounce chicken breast with skin contains about 16 grams of fat. Remove the skin, and that same serving drops to only about 5 grams of fat. Big difference! Thus, removing the poultry skin from your diet makes a significant impact on the amount of fat you consume.

Here's the other great thing about chicken and turkey meat: When ground up, it can often be used as a substitute for the much higher fat ground beef. Ground turkey, especially, is very easy to find in your local grocery store, and typically yields the same low-fat benefits as turkey or chicken breast.

When reading the labels on ground poultry, though watch for the code words.

What you want to buy must be labeled "ground turkey breast" or "ground chicken breast." That guarantees you're getting only lean, healthy white meat in your package. If it doesn't say "breast" or "white meat only" it's a waste of your time.

Why is that important? Well, if you buy a package that just says "ground turkey" or "ground chicken," that means they included white meat, dark meat, and skin when grinding up your purchase—which increases your fat content to about 15 percent of the total.

Way too much for you to get any "fridge benefits" out of it. So insist on the word "breast" on the package.

Other kinds of poultry are a mixed bag, and not often carried in the chain grocery stores, so I don't worry too much about them. However, if something shows up in your store and it looks tasty, check the fat count and give it the same "Extra Lean" test you gave to red meat. Does it come in at about 5 grams of fat or less per serving? Great, enjoy. Higher than five grams per serving? Move along, nothing to see here.

Pork and Lamb

Pig meat and lamb meat are also popular in the local grocery store, but neither of these is generally a good choice. Typically, lamb and pork both carry higher-fat contents more in line with red meats, even though they're considered "light" meats.

There are "lean" cuts of lamb, but I'm not aware of any "extra lean" cuts—and that makes it a difficult choice for your eating plan. Since I come from a middle-eastern background, I ate a lot of lamb growing up. Now that I'm grown and can make my own decisions, I finally just eliminated lamb completely from my diet—one of the few total eliminations in my eating style. I'm not going to say you have to do the same, but I am going to say you'll probably be happier if you do. Still, if you find a cut of lamb that tastes great and comes in at less than five grams of fat per serving, let me know. If it passes the "extra lean" test, I'll be happy to add it back in.

Ham, sausage, bacon—all that kind of stuff you associate with a country breakfast will kill you, and make you suffer on the way. Pepperoni, Canadian bacon, and pizza toppings like that are also deadly for you. Basically, if you want something like that, and it's made from pork, get over it. You should avoid those things completely if you care about your body.

If you like the flavor of foods like bacon or pepperoni (which I do), then be smart and eat the turkey substitutes instead. Again, these taste great, without threatening to give your body a heart attack from fat overload. In fact, Turkey Pepperoni is pretty easy—you only get 4 grams of fat out of 16 or 17 pepperoni slices, which is plenty for pizza topping or calzones or sandwiches or skillet breakfasts and so on.

One caution, though: When buying something like turkey bacon, be sure to check the Nutrition Label because the amount of fat in lean turkey bacon can fluctuate, depending on the manufacturer. For instance, two slices of Jennie-O brand two slices of Jennie-O "lean" turkey bacon contain 5 grams of fat—almost my full fat allowance for breakfast. That's usually OK if I'm having egg-white omelet with sourdough toast or something like that. Still, other brands of turkey bacon may have anywhere from 1.5 grams of fat to 3.0 grams. So, be sure to check the Nutrition Label on your turkey bacon, and in the words of the immortal knight from *Indiana Jones and the Last Crusade*, "Choose wisely."

If you're a big fan of pig, then pork chops or pork tenderloins might be a reasonable option for you. Check the fat content per serving, and trim any visible fat you see, and you'll probably get close to 5 or 6 grams of fat per serving on very lean cuts. But be warned, it's not going to be a lot of actual meat. So be sure to crowd your plate with additional fruits and vegetables so you won't feel hungry after eating it.

Eggs-Cellent!

Now we can move from meat proteins to some of the other categories.

One great source of protein for men is found in eggs. I'm a big fan of eggs, probably because I have many great memories of my grandfather taking me out to breakfast with him when I was a child. We always got the same thing: three eggs, toast, and juice. Good times.

A single egg doesn't contain overmuch in the way of fat—one "large" egg typically holds about 5 grams. The only problem is that one egg is rarely enough food for a man like you and like me. For that reason, if you choose to eat a whole egg be sure to pair it with plenty of other very-low-fat or no-fat accessories like an onion bagel or a big bowl of fruit.

Also, be aware that all of the fat in an egg is in the yolk, so it's extremely easy to eliminate fat completely from the egg equation. Joy! Breakfast just got fun again!

Eating egg-white only is a great, gourmet way to spice up your egg dishes. Simply separate the yolk from the white (crack the egg into your hand and let the white seep through your fingers), dispose of the yolk, and cook up the white.

When eating egg dishes, you can use two egg whites in place of one whole egg. Also, I know of some people who like to mix several egg whites with one whole egg to get the benefit of yolk flavor and color without sacrificing the "fridge benefits" of eating. For instance, they might mix four egg whites with one whole egg for the equivalent of a three-egg omelet. If you like to do that, it's fine, but in my opinion it's really unnecessary. After all, why add fat to food—even healthy food—if you don't need to add it? Still, it's your call on that one.

I also like purchase liquid egg substitute that comes in small cartons. Egg Beaters® is probably the most popular brand name for these, but they also come in generic brands that are essentially the same, but cheaper.

Liquid egg substitutes like Egg Beaters are awesome because they're made from real eggs, they contain no fat and no cholesterol, but are still a good source of daily protein. Basically, products like Egg Beaters are made from egg whites with some food coloring added to give it the look of scrambled eggs or omelets with yolk in. Best of all? Because they're made with real eggs, they taste like eggs—delicious. I eat these eggs all the time, and would happily recommend that you do the same.

You can use liquid egg substitutes as a meal unto themselves, or in any recipe that calls for eggs. Simply measure the amount given on the product (usually 1/4 to 1/3 of a cup) and add this to your recipe. Egg substitutes can also be used for omelets, scrambled eggs, quiches and anything else your creative mind can dream up.

So enjoy eggs all you want—just be sure you take the egg without the fat.

Fish

I hate fish. Even the smell of fish—cooked or raw—sickens me. Can't stand it. In fact, my version of hell is a seafood restaurant (with country music playing and cats as waiters). I figure anything that swims in its own feces should never enter my mouth ... but I digress.

My point is ... I hate fish. But my unrelenting disgust for it is irrelevant because fish is actually a great option for you and your *Dude You Don't Have to Be Fat* lifestyle.

In fact, the American Heart Association recommends that you eat at least two servings of fish each week, especially fish that contains heart-healthy omega-3 fatty acids (such as salmon, tuna, and halibut). [57] And why wouldn't they? Research shows that "in 16 of the 20 countries with the lowest rates of heart disease, people consumed significantly higher quantities of fish." Truth is, fish contains "high-quality protein, healthy unsaturated fats [and] few, if any saturated fats." [58]

So, if you can stomach it, go ahead and indulge your fish itch. In fact, I encourage you to do so (just don't invite me over for dinner when you do).

Generally speaking, medium and dark-fleshed fish (such as salmon and tuna) are a little higher in fat—but they also contain plenty of that precious omega-3—so I'd say to eat them sparingly.

Lighter, white-fleshed fish (such as tilapia, flounder, and cod) brings most of the same benefits as extra lean, white-meat poultry: Very low fat content, high protein and even some omega-3s to boost your system. That sounds like a win all the way around. (Except, or course, you're eating fish.)

Still, as with all protein sources we discussed in this chapter, always—always—check the fat content before buying any fish. Make sure, no matter what it is, that it meets the "Extra Lean" standard we discussed earlier (about 5 grams of fat per serving or less). This is especially true if you're buying shellfish (such as clams, crabs, lobster, etc.). Check the label, Dude. It could save your life.

Dry Beans, Nuts, and Seeds

Beans, nuts, and seeds are the last foodstuffs we'll look at in this chapter. These are the plant alternatives to the other protein foods in this category. When beans are combined with a grain or with a dairy product, they form a complete protein, so meats are not required to maintain a healthy diet that includes protein. Thus a plate of black beans and rice flavored with onions, peppers, and tomatoes, is a low fat meal that's very filling, and still contains the protein your body needs.

Nuts and seeds have protein as well, and since they're plant-based the fat in them is at least one that's better for your body. But nuts are very high in fat. A handful of 14 large cashews has almost 13 grams of fat; one measly tablespoon of chopped pecans has 5 grams of fat (about the same as 8 ounces of chicken breast!), and one tablespoon of chopped peanuts has 4.5 grams of fat. Almonds have less fat than these (just under 4 grams for a tablespoon) and are usually not cooked in additional oil so if you do eat nuts they're a better choice.

The problem, as I'm sure you can see, is that small amounts of nuts have high concentrations of fat. It's really easy to snack too much on nuts—even two moderate handfuls will load your body with unneeded fat grams. I've found it's easiest just to leave nuts out of my *Dude, You Don't Have to be Fat* equation, and would recommend the same for you. The only exception would be when nuts are used sparingly as a garnish or crumbled up for a bit of added flavor and crunch to a larger menu item (such as a salad or an extra lean version of Kung Pao Chicken).

Sad to say, that also includes nut spreads like peanut butter or almond butter. Honestly, guys, there's just too much fat in that stuff—and it's too easy to pile on when eating toast or a PB&J sandwich. Even just two tablespoons of reduced fat peanut butter (barely enough to cover your bread) has a whopping 12 grams of fat in it.

There are one or two peanut butter substitutes that are much lower in fat. For instance, I've occasionally enjoyed the brand product, Better 'N' Peanut Butter, which is made from peanut flour instead of actual peanuts. It has a very peanut-buttery consistency, and while not as strong in flavoring, it is enough let you know you're eating peanut butter. And, best of all, two tablespoons of Better 'N' Peanut Butter holds only two grams of fat (yay!). I've made peanut butter cookies using Better 'N' Peanut Butter, and they weren't bad. Not like Mama used to make, but not bad either. Still, good luck finding that stuff at Walmart or Safeway. It's usually only sold at specialty grocery stores like Trader Joe's or Sprouts, and it's kind of expensive (about six bucks for a small jar).

I'd recommend that you walk away from peanut butter and other nut spreads, at least for now. It's just easier, and it reduces the risk that you'll overdo it next time you want a

PB fix. Remember, you want make it easy to eat well, and keeping high fat nuts and nut spreads within close reach actually sabotages that part of your fight SMART strategy.

All right!

Now that you've conquered the protein-source foods in your grocery store, it's time to tackle dairy and grain products. Ready?

Turn the page and let's keep moving.

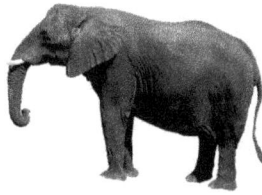

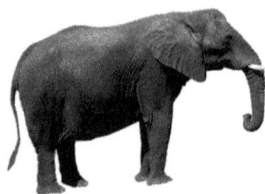

Eleven:

Shopping for Dairy

There are two kinds of stupid in the world.

The first is Ignorant-Stupid, like the people who opt for The Cotton Ball Diet. These morons "begin each meal with an appetizer of cotton balls." They figure cotton balls fill up your stomach so you won't eat too much real food. Stupid! Or the lazy-minded folks who go for The Sleeping Beauty diet, where you take drugs to knock yourself into a temporary coma because, hey, you can't eat while you're sleeping, right? [59] Stupid? Yes, clearly. But Ignorant-Stupid; these people just don't seem to know any better.

The second kind of stupid is Stubborn-Stupid. These are guys who know better, yet act like morons anyway. Take Jordan Lazelle, for instance. Every night, good ol' Jordy insisted on giving a bedtime kiss to his pet ... scorpion. Surprise! One night when he leaned in for a smooch, the scorpion grabbed his lip, jumped into his mouth, and stung him on the tongue—sending Jordan to the hospital for an extended stay. [60] Or take any of the idiots who actually follow the instructions of The Tapeworm Diet: "Travel to a part of the world where beef tapeworms are endemic [and] take one orally." [61]

Stupid, stupid, stoopid.

Stubborn-Stupid is pathetic, so pay attention to what I'm about to say next:

Any guy who eats or drinks any dairy product with fat in it is just as dumb as Jordan Lazelle or a Tapeworm dieter.

Dairy Delights

Look, dairy products like milk, cheese, sour cream, yogurt, cottage cheese, and so on have lots of benefits for you. These kinds of foods provide calcium, vitamins A, B12, and D, potassium, protein, and other nutrients your body needs. Dairy products are so important, in fact, that the USDA recommends that every American have a minimum of three servings of it every single day.

Plus, come on, this stuff tastes great! I mean really, what kind of world with this be if we couldn't eat gourmet grilled cheese sandwiches (see page 211) or banana chocolate milk-shakes (page 156) or ice cream cones or even Cap'n Crunch drowned in cold, fresh milk?

So yes, if you're pursuing a *Dude, You Don't Have to be Fat* path in your life, you should definitely make dairy products a big part of that. But with very few, minor exceptions, you should never—never—consume any milk product that has fat in it. You don't have to do it, so why would you? Here are the facts about milk and milk products:

• Removing fat from milk does NOT remove any nutrients from it. Skim milk (or "fat-free" milk) delivers just as much health benefit as any milk with fat in it does. [62]

• Skim milk actually has the highest concentration of calcium of any milk. This is because calcium is contained in the non-fat part of milk—meaning an 8 ounce glass of skim milk delivers about 306 milligrams of calcium while the same serving of whole milk delivers only 276 milligrams. [63]

Do you see what that means? Fat-free (skim) dairy products give you every good thing about milk products—and none of the harmful fat calories. Dude, that's like going to a bank and getting free money. In fact, in nutritional terms, it's so much like stealing there ought to be a law against it. Lucky for you and me there's not.

"Hey Mikey," you might be saying to me now, "yeah, I hear you on this one. Whole milk—bad. Got it. That's why I drink 2 percent fat milk ... or 1 percent fat milk. Yeh, knock out the fat, right?"

Dude, now you're just being Stubborn-Stupid again.

Didn't you hear what I said?

Nutritionally speaking, fat-free milk has everything whole milk, or 2 percent milk, or 1 percent milk has. So why would you want to waste your allowable fat grams today on something that's unnecessary? Even more, why would you bother consuming any amounts of harmful fat in your dairy products when you could be getting ZERO amounts of fat instead?

Look, imagine I made you a choice of these three offers:

1) Meet me tomorrow and I'll give you $100.
2) Meet me tomorrow and I'll give you $100 along with five punches in the nose.
3) Meet me tomorrow and I'll give you $100 along with two punches in the nose.

Seriously, which of those offers are you going to take? It's a no-brainer, right? You'll take the hundred bucks and ZERO punches in the nose. So why wouldn't you use the same line of reasoning in your choice of dairy products? Basically, your dairy universe is offering you the same three choices with nutrition and fat. You can:

1) Consume fat-free milk products and get health benefits with no fat-punches to body.
2) Consume 2 percent fat milk and get health benefits along with 5 fat-punches (about 5 grams of fat) to your body.
3) Consume 1 percent fat milk and get health benefits plus 2 1/2 fat-punches (about 2 1/2 grams of fat) to your body.

What do you think is the best choice? You know the answer, so stop whining and make the smart choice.

Shopping for Dairy

With that in mind, shopping for dairy products is extremely easy:

Always get the fat-free option.

There, it's simple as that.

Now, the USDA doesn't categorize cream cheese, cream, and butter as part of the dairy food group because they say the calcium content is not significant. That's their problem. As far as *Dude, You Don't Have to be Fat* is concerned, "dairy" refers to any product made from milk. So, when you're shopping for dairy at your grocery store, the "fat-free" rule should apply to anything in the dairy section (such as milk, yogurt, cheese, sour cream, cottage cheese, cream cheese, buttermilk and so on) as well as any dairy desserts or dairy cooking products (such as milkshakes, ice cream, frozen yogurt, pudding, evaporated milk, whipped cream, half-n-half, and the like).

At first it may seem to you that fat-free milk is less substantial, or "watery" than the milk you've been used to. Get over it. It only takes about one to two weeks for your taste buds (and your subconscious expectations) to adjust to the new consistency, and then you'll never notice it again. Yogurt, sour cream, coffee creamer, cottage cheese, and most other dairy products that are fat free taste almost exactly the same as the high-fat versions, so those should be easy for you.

I've found that fat-free cheese comes in both shredded and sliced packages at your local Walmart, and occasionally at your Kroger store. It's also available in both cheddar and mozzarella, so pizzas and sandwiches and cheese sauces and pretty much everything you love about cheese is still available to you in fat-free form.

Sprouts Farmers Markets and Whole Foods grocery chains also carry "Lifetime" brand (http://www.lifetimecheese.com) of block cheeses in the following fat-free varieties: Cheddar, Sharp Cheddar, Swiss, Monterey Jack, Jalapeño Jack, Garden Vegetable, Mild Mexican, and Mozzarella. These are delicious! Get them if you can. If you don't have Sprouts or Whole Foods in your area, you can still order all varieties of Lifetime fat free cheeses online from Northwoods Cheese Company at: http://www.northwoodscheese.com/LifetimeCheese.html.

Be sure to look for the words "Fat Free" on your cheese purchases. At first these cheeses may seem to be not as "sharp," or strong as fat-filled cheese, but again, it only takes a little bit of time of consistent usage for your taste buds to adjust. And if you're tempted to go back to fat-filled cheeses, remember: "cheese contains about *six times the amount* of saturated fat than found in beef tenderloin" [64] (italics mine). That's a lot of fat! Don't bother with it. Instead, eat gobs of fat-free cheese and enjoy it. Even if you decided to "double-cheese" to flavor your pizza, you're still not getting any fat, so have at it.

Occasionally, I've found that Walmart and/or Kroger may not carry the fat-free mozzarella in every market or in all four seasons, though I don't have a clue as to why. For instance, recently I found Kraft fat-free mozzarella in a Walmart in Oklahoma, but the next day at my home Walmart store in Colorado, it was not in stock. Go figure. If that happens to you when you're making pizza, you can substitute Kraft low-moisture, part skim mozzarella instead. Because this is made from 2% milk, it does contain some fat, so use only 3/4 cup of the part-skim mozzarella, and mix in a little fat-free cheddar if you like that taste. Doing this adds 12 grams of fat to your entire pizza, which should be fine since it's spread over 8 slices of (adding only about 1.5 grams of fat per slice). Still, use this as your back-up option as fat-free mozzarella is always the better choice, if it's available.

Feta cheese and Roquefort (bleu) cheeses are others that are typically used in recipes in small amounts only as a seasoning or flavor tip—not as a main dish or a main snack. As such, they can be reasonable additions to your *Dude, You Don't Have to be Fat* plan as long as you're careful. HOWEVER, remember to moderate your use of any these cheeses, and to count the fat grams as part of your daily intake. If you do that, you'll be fine.

By the way, Feta cheese does come in a fat-free version, but I only find it at my Walmart in the summertime. Again, I have no idea why. Still you might want to look for it first if you need Feta for some recipe.

Parmesan cheese already tends to be lower in fat, but I haven't found a fat-free option for it at my local Walmart. That makes this cheese one of your extremely rare exceptions to "exclusively fat-free dairy" rule. Because it's used mostly as just seasoning with other foods it's generally not a big deal.

A Bit about Butter

Butter is the only other minor exception to this totally fat-free rule—but that's only when it comes to baking, not to everyday butter consumption.

Truth is, fat-free butter or margarine is nearly impossible to find at your local Walmart or Kroger store, even though several companies make it. I Can't Believe It's Not Butter! brand of products has a fat-free "soft-spread" that tastes nice and buttery. Promise brand margarines also has a fat-free spread that's fine. And Smart Beat brand has a fat-free option in their squeeze bottle margarines. But, again, good luck finding these in basic grocery stores like Walmart or Safeway.

If you can get one of the fat-free butter spreads at your local grocery, then you should. Ask your customer service team at your local store, or check online to find it. But if you can't, then you'll probably want to go with the I Can't Believe It's Not Butter! spray bottle.

This is like liquid butter (though much less dense) and has a fine buttery taste to it. I use it for topping on toast and rolls, all kinds of breads, vegetables, as well as for flavoring when cooking potatoes and eggs in a skillet. It's versatile and great for most butter options—and Walmart even carries a generic brand of this, so it's pretty inexpensive and easy to find. You can also buy Butter Buds in the spice aisle, which helps flavor food the same way salt and pepper do, but with dried, buttery flakes instead. Personally, I like the buttery spray better, but give both a try and see which you find more appealing.

When it comes to baking, however, sometimes a little bit of butter is required to make the bakery item hold together. Yes, there are several substitutes for butter than can be used in most baking (such as applesauce, cream cheese, and Sunsweet brand's Lighter Bake), and it's always best to use those for recipes if you can. So you won't often need any real butter—except for some baking projects. When that happens, always choose the lightest fat butter product, and always use less than the recipe asks for (using a majority of the butter substitute). And then make sure you calculate the fat content per servings so that no single serving has more fat in it than you will allow.

Still, except for that minor exception in baking, you really never need any dairy product that has fat in it—so make it your habit never to buy anything besides fat-free milk products.

OK, I think you're ready. Now, let's get into grains...

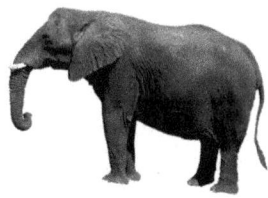

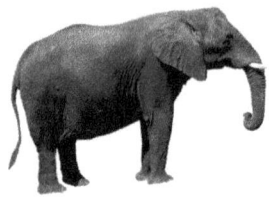

Twelve:
Shopping for Grain-Based Foods

The "Grains" food group covers quite a bit of ground.

A grain-based food is anything made from wheat, rice, oats, cornmeal, barley, or another cereal grain. This includes foods such as breads, cereals, crackers, pasta, oatmeal, rice, muffins, tortillas, pitas, flatbreads, and even desserts like cake and pie crusts.

In other words, the Grain food group is awesome.

"Grains are the world's most plentiful food," says Dr. William Sears, "and enjoy first place in the diet of nearly every culture." Grains are a superb source of protein, complex carbohydrates, fiber, zinc, iron, folic acid, minerals, and B vitamins—all of which are necessary to keep that body of yours running well. "And there's more great news about grains," says Dr. Sears. "They're naturally low in fat." [65]

Like I said, awesome.

What's crazy is that grains are where many fad diets cut people off, saying we should avoid grains like breads, rice, and pasta. That's just bull's pizzle.

These are the foods that give us a feeling of being full, and that offer so many nutrients our bodies need. And since they're naturally low-fat, we can eat a lot of them (unless they've been fattened up with oils or higher-fat fillings and toppings).

For instance, in a typical day I could stuff myself with a few bowls of cereal for breakfast, a bagel for a mid-morning snack, a sandwich for lunch, a roll with dinner, and a bowl of low-fat popcorn later in the evening. That's a lot of food—and it's all low fat. With that much tasty variety available to me in the Grain food group every day, it's practically impossible that I'm going to go hungry anytime soon.

However, we do need to be aware that the more "processed" grains are, the more they lose nutrients. Since you and I need all the good stuff we can get, look for products that use whole grains, and that have the fewest additives. Whole grains (like wheat and oat and brown rice) contain the entire grain kernel and therefore provide full nutritional value.

For some reason, we've misnamed weakened, processed grain foods as "enriched." They say all marketers are liars, and this is proof. Enriched grains show up in products like white bread, white flour, cakes, some cereals and the like. Any product with "enriched" grain has been "refined" in a factory where it was bleached and processed for easier consumption and a supposedly more attractive appearance. As part of that "enriching" process, essential nutrients such as thiamin, riboflavin, niacin, and iron have been forcibly removed from your food. [66] I know, Stubborn-Stupid.

The point is, even if it's low fat, you're probably better off avoiding "enriched" grain foods, or at least cutting back on them. The common-sense approach put forth by the USDA says to make at least 50 percent of the grain foods you eat ones that benefit from "whole grain" preparation. That sounds reasonable to me.

Also, with all foods in this group, be aware that simply being grain-based doesn't mean something is inherently low-fat.

Our society has become quite adept at taking healthy grain foods and transforming them into unconstitutional junk. For instance, doughnuts are a grain-based food, but the recipes for preparing them add in enormous amounts of unhealthy fat and sugars that can—literally—kill you. Hey, there's a reason why the prevailing stereotype of "fat police officer" is the one where they all sit around eating doughnuts. So be aware of how your grain foods have been prepared (Baked? Yes! Fried? No!) and what kinds of other ingredients have been added to your grain foods. After all, you don't want to be mistaken for a fat cop, do you?

Buy Grains that Fit Your Fat Intake Standards

Regardless of what kind of grain food you're buying, be sure to check the Nutrition Facts label to see what the fat content is. Make sure that eating that food will fit within the boundaries you've set for your daily allowance of fat intake. That's your golden rule for buying grain-based foods.

For instance, if you plan on having sandwiches for lunch while you're at work this week, don't buy the bread that packs 3.5 grams of fat into every slice. If you do that, then the grain alone in your lunch each day would hit 7 grams. Instead, buy the bread that holds only 1 gram of fat per slice. That way, your grains only contribute 2 grams total to your lunch, and you can fill out the rest of your lunch allowance of fat with good stuff to go between the bread slices. Make sense?

As part of your diligent nutrition check, also be sure you look at the serving size.

For example, a large muffin you grab from the vending machine at work may actually be so large that it counts as two or more servings. Read the label on the side of a package to see how much of the product the manufacturer has identified as one serving. If you're going to eat more than that, figure your fat counts accordingly.

In general, one slice of bread is a serving. That means, unless it says differently on the package, a hamburger bun or sandwich roll (which has both a top slice and a bottom slice) is two servings. Same goes for a pita. One cup of packaged cereal (like corn flakes) is a serving, and ½ a cup of rice, pasta, or cooked cereals (like oatmeal) is a serving. One tortilla is usually only one serving as well. You get the idea.

Now let's dig into specific grain foods a little bit more.

Breads

When you shop for loaves of bread at the grocery store, you'll find a number of breads with a "low-fat" label. Unfortunately, too many of these are flimsy bits of mush with no real substance. In fact, some of these are very similar in content to regular white bread, and have just been cut into thinner slices so that the fat per serving is less.

However, take heart. You can still find breads made with whole grains that are tasty, filling, and don't have a lot of added oil. Whole wheat bread is usually a good choice, unless it has been flavored with fatty ingredients (check the label!). Sourdough bread is one of my favorites, and is almost always low in fat. Plus, it's dense enough to be filling (and not to fall apart when you add a few slices of lunchmeat, tomato and cucumber between two pieces).

Our family has also found delicious, low-fat breads at the bakery inside the supermarket. We purchase several loaves at a time and store them in the freezer. The bakery often uses freshly ground wheat and other grains, sweetens with honey instead of sugar and oil, and doesn't add unwanted preservatives. Talk to bakery employees to find out what your options are there. You might also find a local independent bakery or franchised quick-service restaurant cooking up some good breads in your neighborhood, so check around. Good bread is out there. (Panera bread is my favorite!)

If you're the chef type, you may also choose to make your own bread. There's nothing like the smell of homemade bread! Bread machines are popular, or you can stick with the "old-fashioned" method of kneading bread by hand. Either way, look for recipes and mixes that use little or no oils so you can enjoy your bread without consuming unwanted fats. My wife has come up with an easy recipe that can be used for loaves of bread or for dinner rolls and such. I stole it from her and included it for you in the "snacks" section of the Mini-Cookbook for Men later in this book (page 153).

Cereals

I'm actually a big fan of cold cereal—something I passed on to my son. When he was a kid, he'd often take a bowl of cereal to school and pour his little carton of milk over it for his lunch. Even now, well into my middle-age years, I eat cereal anytime of the day. I'll snack on it dry, right out the box, sneak it into movie theaters, and even take a sandwich baggie full of it with me when I'm running errands around town. With skim milk added, I also like eat it for a frequent nighttime snack. It fills me up and helps me sleep with a comfortably full stomach all night long.

Cereal tastes good, is filling, and is fortified with all kinds of vitamins. (It could be just hearsay, but I've even heard that cold cereal has become the number one source of vitamins for children in America.) Plus, it's often very low in fat. In fact, there are dozens of options on my cereal aisle that sport only one gram or 1.5 grams of fat in a bowl. Since I like to eat about three servings of cereal at a sitting, that works out to between 3 to 4.5 grams of fat for my morning meal—perfect for my breakfast fat intake on a normal day. Hard to go wrong with that!

If you also like cold cereal, look for ones that are high in fiber, and low in sugar and fat. Be careful of some of the "health food" cereals such as granola, as these are often baked in oils and will actually be very fatty. In fact, one box I saw at Walmart recently showed that a half a cup of a certain brand of granola had 10 grams of fat! That's criminal! A guy like you or like me should be able to eat hearty grains without someone pouring fat on top of them. So look for the companies that make cereals without the added fat

Hot cereals (like oatmeal or cream of wheat) are generally low in fat and high in fiber and nutrients. They also tend to be filling and satisfying when you're hungry. Good stuff. My wife actually keeps a few packets of instant oatmeal at her desk. If she gets hungry for something warm and filling while at work, she just adds a little water in her mug, zaps it in the microwave, and she's got a satisfying snack in minutes. If you work in an office environment, that could be a good idea for you too.

Rice and Pasta

Rice and pasta also provide nutrients guys like us need, and they give a satisfying feeling of being full. Most people don't like these foods plain, so rice and pasta are often cooked with oils or are covered with gravies or sauces. That's a shame—and it's unnecessary.

There are many ways to prepare rice and pasta so these foods will taste great, but without all the added fat. Try preparing rice or pasta in fat-free chicken or vegetable broth. Or cook it plain, and add dry seasonings like lemon-pepper or garlic and herbs. Better yet, eat brown rices or low-fat wild rices that have flavor built right in.

At any rate, as long as they don't have unnecessary added fats, these grains are great for your plate—particularly whole grain versions of them. So always keep a few extra boxes of rice or pasta in your pantry, and pull them out frequently to add to your meals.

Other Grains

Other grain-based foods include tortillas, dinner rolls, muffins, corn bread, and more. The list of foods made with grains goes on and on—and it's all good. Just remember to always look for any "hidden fat" in these foods, either in added ingredients or ridiculously small "serving size" amounts. For example, store-bought muffins are usually very high in fat. Croissants are also fat hogs that'll kill you.

Be aware, too, that tortillas made with white flour and butter are heavy in fat (and totally unnecessary). Just about every brand of tortilla maker has some version of a "low fat" or "heart healthy" tortilla, so reach for that package and ignore all the others. I personally like the Mission brand "96 percent Fat Free Medium/Soft Taco Tortillas." These taste every bit as good as a full-fat tortilla, but carry only 1.5 grams of fat per tortilla. That's a win for everybody. Olé Mexican Foods brand also makes an "extreme wellness" fat-free tortilla that's suitable for south-of-the-border dishes. Corn tortillas are often low in fat too, and can be a good option for you in this regard.

Be aware, however, that unless they're baked, even a small bag of corn tortilla chips can pack on the fat grams.

I love nachos, so recently I was checking for healthy options in corn chips. I already had my bag of fat-free cheese in the cart, just needed the chips to go with it. I found a bag of tortilla chips at my grocery store that had a "low-fat" label on them. They looked tasty with special spices on them, so I turned the bag over to see how much fat was in one serving. Only 3 grams per serving—looking good. Then I checked to see how big the serving was. Eight chips. Eight chips? I can eat that in two bites!

Nearby was another bag of tortilla chips that also claimed to be low in fat. I checked out that label and found that these chips also only had 3 grams of fat per serving. This time the serving was 18 chips—enough to fill an entire nacho plate. Quite a difference! Reading labels allowed me to eat enough chips to feel like I'd actually had a snack, without adding unwanted grams of fat. You'd be wise to do the same.

Another option is for you just to oven-make your own tortilla chips. It's actually fairly easy, and (if you do it right!) it tastes pretty good. It just takes time and effort to make your own chips, so I've always found it easier just to buy the low-fat, baked bag at the grocery store. Still, if you're interested in oven-baking your own tortilla chips, do a quick Internet search for "homemade tortilla chip recipe" and you should find what you need. Just make sure you exclude butter and oil from any recipe you find. Give it a try, you might like it.

All right, now you know how to conquer the grain-based products in your local grocery store and kitchen! Toss out the fatty croissants, lame corn chips, and heavy-fat granolas.

Dude, You Don't Have to be Fat

Restock your shelves with hearty breads, baked chips, and plenty of lower fat cereals. Stock up on oatmeal, rice, and pasta. You'll enjoy eating a lot of these foods.

Now we're off to dominate fruit and vegetables. See you in the next chapter!

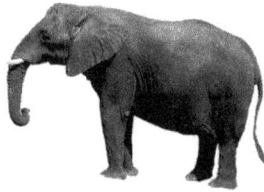

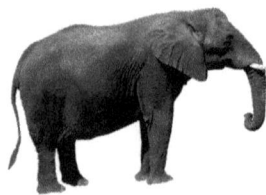

Thirteen:
Shopping for Produce

When my son, Tony, was young, he went grocery shopping with me or my wife every week.

From a child's point of view, the grocery store was a marvelous place. Brightly colored packages, cartoon character faces popping off of every container. Promises of toys inside boxes. So much to look at and so much to buy! Tony, like many children, began to develop a habit of asking for just about anything he saw at the grocery store.

"Can we buy that cereal? Can I have that candy? I want some of those! Let's buy that!"

My wife and I always felt like villains saying, "No" all the time. First of all, we simply couldn't afford to buy everything Tony wanted. And second, a lot of the things he asked for were just junk. Amy and I wanted Tony to love good foods, not junk.

One day Amy hit upon an idea that changed everything. As they rounded the corner to the produce section of the grocery store, she spread her arms to the vast array of colorful fruits and vegetables.

"Tony," she said, "You can choose anything you want from this area. Every week you can choose anything you want, and as much as you want, from this area and we'll buy it."

Tony was about four at the time, and he smiled his most endearing smile. He jumped off the end of the cart and began exploring. Over the coming weeks and months and years he chose a wide variety of foods he'd previously turned up his nose at, like Brussels sprouts and asparagus and cauliflower. And he got our whole family to try foods we'd never even heard of, like carambola fruit and Bosc pears. Thanks to Tony, over the years I've eaten eggplant (not great, not terrible), an array of squashes (I don't like 'em, but my wife thinks they're great), oranges from other countries (delicious!), apples of all colors, kumquats, snow peas, plantains, and persimmons. We've had to hunt down store employees who can tell us the names of these foods—and then how to eat or prepare them. And through it all it was a great adventure.

Sometimes, after shopping with his mom, Tony would come home with a bag of some crazy new fruit or vegetable and show it off to me. (I'd try not to give a look of horror when I saw yet another kind of squash.)

"Look what I picked out!" he'd say to me with genuine enthusiasm. So we all ate it, whatever it was, and discovered that most of it was actually pretty darn good. Tony is grown and married now, and still willing to try new foods because of this childhood approach to buying fruits and vegetables.

Funny thing happened after Tony moved out, though. I started missing that weekly fruit-or-vegetable surprise. So even today, whenever I turn the corner into the produce aisle at Walmart or King Soopers, I pause just to take in the spectacle of deliciousness before me. My eyes start glittering, and pretty soon I'm the four-year-old kid dumping all kinds of exciting new options into our shopping cart.

You see, our whole family had learned to try new fruits and vegetables this way, and unexpectedly, it became a joyful way of life for all of us. In the process, it also opened our eyes to the wide array of fruits and vegetables available these days. Gone are the days when apples and oranges were the only fruit options, and corn and green beans were the only vegetables on the table. There's a whole world of produce goodness out there, fellas. It's time we took advantage of that.

So here's your rule for shopping in the produce section:
Any fruit or vegetable you see, you can buy.

Easy, huh? And fun. When you and your family are shopping in the produce section, give yourself permission to buy any fruit or any vegetable you want from that area—and buy as much as you want. (Okay, there are two notable exceptions to this rule, but we'll get to those shortly. Meanwhile...)

If you need to dump other stuff to make room in your cart (or your budget), do it. Pack your grocery bags with enough fruits and vegetables to pack your kitchen with great fruit and vegetable options all week long.

Next, begin experimenting with your produce buys. Try a fruit you've never eaten before. Grate or chop vegetables into your casseroles. Keep bowls of fruit on your counter. Select some produce whose name you can't pronounce. Carry bags of snow peas, sliced peppers, and cherry tomatoes along to the office—veggies are great for snacking since they're so low in calories, nearly fat-free, and full of nutrients. You can offer them to yourself and your family at any time. Steam vegetables or serve them raw. Offer fruit as a salad or a dessert. Raid your spice cabinet and experiment with different seasonings.

Oh, and don't forget about liquid fruit and veggies! Choose 100 percent fruit or vegetable juices instead of soft drinks—and enjoy tasty, thirst-quenching drinks that have all the benefits of your grocery store's produce aisle. Good call, bro!

Why So Fruity, Mikey?

My son used to call fruit "God's candy," and I think it's true. These foods are good raw or cooked, and fruit has a natural sugar (fructose or sucrose) that makes it sweet without any of the harmful side effects of processed sweeteners.

Hey, there's a reason why so many candies and desserts are fruit-flavored—it's cuz those fruits are already sweet and delicious like dessert. As Charlie Sheen would say: Winning!

The amazing thing with fruits and vegetables is how good they are for you. I'm always finding studies showing how eating more apples, broccoli, or leafy vegetables, or more of anything from this food group has been found to lengthen life, give more energy, lower the chances of getting cancer, and on and on. This stuff is great for you, and with such a wide variety of choices, it's nearly impossible not to find some kind of produce you'll love to eat.

Fruit is typically packed with vitamin C, antioxidants, enzymes, and soluble fiber that your body needs. Thanks to its natural sugars, fruit also delivers a natural energy boost. Dr. William Sears reports, "Fructose is absorbed slowly into the bloodstream, so fruit gives you energy without triggering the ups and downs of the insulin cycle." [67]

Fruits and vegetables also deliver essential minerals and additional, necessary vitamins that keep your body running at peak performance. Plus, vegetables and fruits have been proven to: help prevent heart disease and stroke; help control blood pressure; help fight certain kinds of cancer; help preserve eyesight and vision; and help your gastrointestinal tract to stay functioning and healthy. [68]

I like the picturesque way that self-proclaimed "skinny bitches," Rory Freedman and Kim Barnouin, describe photosynthesis and the fantastic effect fruits and vegetables provide for your bag of bones:

> Plants store the sun's energy, which we receive by eating them. If you can, just picture the light energy from the sun beaming down to the vegetables and fruits, and as we eat those foods, imagine that energy being transmitted into our bodies. Our nervous systems are maintained and stimulated by this light. What an amazing gift from nature—to be able to eat such pure foods that give our bodies so much. [69]

Hard to argue against that. It's no wonder, then, that the USDA recommends you fill half your plate at every meal with fruits and vegetables. With *Dude, You Don't Have to be Fat*, I recommended going even further. In addition to enjoying fruit and veggies at every meal, keep loads of the stuff conveniently located in your kitchen and at your workplace so you can enjoy it as a snack anytime, anywhere you are during a day.

And like I said before, remember that fruit and vegetables can be drunk as well as eaten. I keep several gallons of fruit juice in my pantry at all times. I'm a big fan of cherry juice and also kiwi-strawberry juice, and my wife like vegetable juice blends like V-8. So drink up—just make sure that the juices you buy are labeled "100 percent fruit juice" or "100 percent vegetable juice." Anything else is just "flavored" with juice or vegetables, and doesn't do much for your body except quench thirst.

You can enjoy fruit as a spread for bread in the form of jams and jellies as well. You can even cook jelly inside rolls for a hot, sticky treat. As with juices, just remember when buying jams and jellies to always buy products labeled "100 percent fruit" instead of some partial fruit mixture.

Unfortunately the only fruit or vegetable some guys eat is the lettuce and tomato that comes on their fast-food burger, along with fat-drenched, fried potatoes that have just about nothing good left in them after being boiled in oil. Open your eyes, Dude, and soon you'll see all the good fruits and vegetables literally spread out before you. In fact, right now I'm looking at a ranking of the "100 Best Health Foods," and the top 20 items on that list are exclusively fruits. Want to guess what item numbers 21-49 are? Yep, vegetables. Starting to see a pattern here? (If not, you're a moron.)

Be aware that fruits and vegetables do have trace amounts of fat in them, but it's often so low it's not worth counting. For example, one cup of diced cantaloupe has 0.2 grams of fat. A cup of raw carrots has 0.1 grams of fat. So you could eat plate after plate of these and still take in only minimal amounts of fat.

One important warning though: **the notable exceptions in the produce aisle are avocados and olives**—so be careful when you choose those for your kitchen. You don't need to avoid them completely, just be careful and be sure to count their fat content against your daily fat intake goals.

One whole avocado averages 30 grams of fat all by itself, so never eat it solo or as a main dish. Use avocado instead the way you would nuts, sparingly and as a seasoning or a garnish for other foods instead of as a snack or a meal itself. For instance, putting one tablespoon of avocado on a sandwich adds only about two and a half grams of fat while spicing up that turkey lunch meat in a delicious way.

Likewise, a serving of only ten olives has between five and seven grams of fat, depending on the type of olive and the size. Again, you'll want to choose olives less often, and when you choose them use them only as garnishes or seasoning, and eat them sparingly.

Other than that, go hog wild, Dude.

I personally am a "fruit anytime," kind of guy. I actually get annoyed when there's no fruit left in the house ... I start craving it like candy. (Yes, I have been known to make a late-night run to the grocery store just to get blackberries for snacking on during halftime of Monday Night Football.) My wife likes fruit, but she loves vegetables. She'll cook up Brussels sprouts just for a snack, and eat raw carrots and broccoli just cuz she thinks they taste good.

You may be somebody who prefers fruits or someone who prefers vegetables. Fine, eat away, bro. Don't purposefully exclude either fruit or vegetables, but hey, feel free to indulge your favorites at the same time.

At the grocery store, load your cart with fresh and frozen fruits and vegetables. The more the better!

At home, keep fruit and vegetables on your counters or washed and ready to eat in the fridge. Let these become your new snack foods.

Keep a few bags of dried fruits in the cabinet—they're so sweet and tasty! Every time you prepare a meal, steam a pan of vegetables or cut slices of fruit and leave these on the table for everyone to enjoy. And be at least as courageous as my four-year-old son—look for some fruit or vegetable you've never tried before and bring it home for a taste test. Ask your produce worker for ideas on how to prepare it, or check the Internet for recipes that use your unique new item. Then see what happens—you might just find your new favorite food.

Okay, one last thought before we exit this chapter. This one comes from nutritionist, Molly Morgan. Through her company, Creative Nutrition Solutions, Molly frequently counsels individual and corporate clients on how to take control of their weight and food health. Naturally, she (like me) is a big advocate of fruiting up your life. She reports, "I'm always shocked to hear the reason why most of my clients aren't getting their daily fill of fruit: They don't keep it in the house. It's practically impossible to eat more fruit without having it on hand." [70]

Don't be as stupid as Molly Morgan's clients. When you hit the produce aisle of your local grocery store, choose any fruit or vegetable that anybody in your family wants from this section. Buy as much as you can eat, and keep it readily at hand in your home every day.

Winning!

Fourteen:
Sugar, Desserts, Alcohol, & Salt

All right! Yesterday you were just another fat guy who mindlessly chugged French fries because they were there. Today you are a lean-machine-in-the-making, a brilliant strategist and your own ally in pursuing the goal of food health for your life.

Way to go, Dude. You rock.

If you've read the last several chapters, you now know how to buy food that'll transform your kitchen into a veritable treasure trove of delicious "fridge benefits" that'll, in turn, transform your body—and your life—into a joyful, comfortable experience.

Now, with the *Dude, You Don't Have to be Fat* approach to eating, there's really no food group that's off limits to you—you just need to be sure to stay within your fat intake goals for each day. At the same time, some food and beverages offer you more benefits than others. We've talked about most of those already. Still, there are a few leftover categories that we should at least address briefly, simply because they can impact your weight and health experience.

Let's tackle those now.

Sugar and Desserts

As has likely been obvious to you, I'm not one of the sugar-haters you so often read about in books like this one.

When I first started changing my eating habits to a *Dude, You Don't Have to be Fat*-friendly style, I didn't bother counting sugar grams or sugar content in my diet. I focused exclusively on daily fat intake. I continued to eat dessert as long as it was low-fat or no-fat. I helped myself to fat-free candies and to low-fat or no-fat ice cream and the like. As you can see, the result in my life after more than a decade has been entirely positive.

A year or two ago, as part of a religious observance, I did go one full month without eating any sugar (except what naturally occurs in fruit). I ate fruit and vegetables only, with no seasoning or other toppings. Because I've read so much about the negative impact of sugar, I was curious to see how that month-long sugar fast would impact my health and daily experience.

In the end—and this is just my own experience, not medical

advice—I didn't notice any real change at all.

My weight stayed the same. My energy level was the same. My general life attitude and health stayed the same. I did notice that I didn't miss sugared sodas as much as I thought I would, so it's possible that some element of a sugar addiction was corrected there, but overall I was actually disappointed by the seeming lack of impact after eliminating sugar completely from my diet.

Still, I think it's important to point out that I was never an "overachiever" in my sugar intake anyway, so it may be that going without sugar completely was not enough of a difference from my regular diet. That could be why I didn't notice any change. Typically, I used to drink one sugared soda a day, and then have one dessert a day (usually cookies or pie or individually-packaged candy and the like). I also ate sugared cereals pretty frequently. But some days I'd forget, or just not be in the mood for it, and not eat much sugar at all, so my experience is kind of a crapshoot here.

Generally speaking, though, we do know that sugar—especially processed or "refined" white sugar—is not a great choice for everyday eating. This is particularly true with packaged, mass-produced, ready-to-eat foods. In fact, in some cases, a manufacturer will increase sugar content in a low-fat product simply because it tastes better—and thus, sells better—that way.

The aforementioned "skinny bitches" even go so far as to declare that "sugar is the devil." "Sugar is like crack," they say, "and food manufacturers know that if they add it to their products, you'll keep coming back for more." [71]

I don't know that I'd go quite that far, but I do want you to recognize that sugar can be dangerous, and can even sabotage your *Dude, You Don't Have to be Fat* goals if you overindulge in that way. You must remember that sugar isn't simply in soda and desserts—it shows up in breads, crackers, pastries, cereals, yogurts, dairy products, frozen breakfast meals, and sometimes even in meat recipes (the Maid-Rite burger comes to mind).

Here's what we know:

Sugar by itself has pretty much no nutritional value. Additionally, according to fitness expert Jackie Warner, "[Sugar] weakens your immune system. It throws off your metabolic functions and is highly addictive." Sugar has also been linked to pancreatic cancer, colon cancer, and stomach cancer. [72] And Dr. Louis Aronne says clearly that, "Sugar is fattening." He points to research studies that illustrate pretty convincingly that sugar's addictive qualities can create an overeating, non-nutritional lifestyle that is difficult to fight, and which leads to heavier, unhealthier bodies. [73]

So, as you can see, too much sugar in your daily diet can be a factor in your weight, and can even interfere with your ability to achieve your goals from a *Dude, You Don't Have to be Fat* lifestyle. At the same time, high sugar content is often paired with higher fat in recipes (i.e. doughnuts or ice cream), so by downsizing your fat intake each day you will naturally also be downsizing your sugar intake.

In the end, you're going to have to make your own call on what's appropriate sugar intake for you. Regardless of what you decide here, be sure that primary goal each day is to lower the fat intake in your diet, knowing that just doing that alone will also significantly lower the amount of sugar you eat each day as well.

Alcohol

Like sugar, alcohol is one of those empty-calorie choices that doesn't easily conform to a hard-and-fast rule.

Now, before we get too far on this topic, for the purposes of the discussion here I'm going to assume that you know the obvious: Anything more than rare to moderate drinking is unhealthy for a host of reasons that include emotional, physical, relational, and spiritual consequences. Particularly any kind of addiction to alcohol is extremely harmful and to be avoided.

My coauthor, Dr. Risenhoover, tells me that the guideline used by dependency counselors to determine if someone is drinking excessively is more than 4 drinks in 24 hours, three times weekly. Additionally, if you have relationship or law enforcement difficulties related to alcohol, then your drinking is problematic and should be curtailed. If that's you, you know it—and you should do something about it.

Still, let's be clear on one thing: I'm not qualified to serve as your twelve-step recovery buddy, so I'm going to assume that you know how to drink responsibly—and that you practice that as well.

With that in mind, I can't see much in the way of benefits from including beer or alcohol in your eating plan.

Men's Health editor-in-chief, David Zinczenko says it well, I think: "It's like funneling excess calories and sugar into your bloodstream to eventually be stored as fat. Think of most drinks as bad TV—time spent with them will likely be a waste." [74]

On the bright side, alcohol has no fat in it. However, it certainly contains calories. Beer has some carbohydrates, obviously an energy (calorie) source. But alcohol itself is metabolized into calories, so a drink like vodka contains no fat, no protein, no carbohydrates, just pure calories that are nutritiously empty and quickly transformed into fat within your body.

According to Dr. Risenhoover, from a nutritional standpoint, drinking alcohol is not much different than consuming sugar—but alcohol has more extreme, potentially hazardous consequences related to behavior, cognitive impairment, and both acute and chronic disease. Alcohol can increase stomach acid production, leading to stomach lining irritation (gastritis), acid reflux disease, even bleeding ulcers. Plus, there is no specific health benefit to drinking beer, so to his mind (and mine), it seems pretty useless to include it in your eating plan.

Additionally, Dr. Kim Bruno reports that "If you're drinking alcohol with food, you're actually perpetuating that whole 'leaky gut' syndrome, where you're not able to break down your food fully... You're getting more diarrhea, more constipation, more bloating, more gas." [75]

Alcohol can also make you feel like you're hungry when your stomach is actually satisfied, and it contributes to obesity "by lessening the body's ability to burn fat. Fat storage is promoted, particularly in the belly—a health danger zone." [76] Additionally, a study at the University of Buffalo in New York showed a clear connection between binge drinking (more than four drinks at a time at least once every two weeks) and abdominal fat. [77]

So if you don't like hauling around that tub of lard you call a belly, you'll probably want to leave alcohol out of your eating (and partying) choices.

What's more, drinking alcohol impairs your decision-making ability, which in turn could tamper with your ability to make good choices for low-fat or no-fat options to eat while you are drinking.

If you still think that alcohol should be an important part of your food consumption, then make wise, moderate choices. Try a glass of red wine for its antioxidant and possible heart health benefits, and limit your drinking to only once or twice per week. Also, since we know that alcohol has an appetite-stimulating effect and that some people have a difficult time losing weight if they drink, Dr. Louis Aronne suggests that the best time to drink alcohol is after a meal—not before. "This is when you'll have the most control," advises Dr. Aronne, and you'll be less likely to make poor food choices, since you are already full. [78]

Personally, I don't drink at all, simply because I don't see any real physical or lifestyle benefit to it. But if you decide to pick up some alcohol during your trip to the grocery store, you're welcome to do so—just monitor your alcohol consumption to be sure it's not sabotaging your personal goals in the *Dude, You Don't Have to be Fat* lifestyle.

Salt/Sodium

Salt has its place in the *Dude, You Don't Have to be Fat* eating plan, and for good reason. Sodium is an important part of your body's physiology, helping nerve function, muscle strength and balancing fluids in your body. Plus, it adds flavor to just about anything, and is a natural preservative for foods. However, we don't really need a lot of salt to get all those benefits—only about one teaspoon (2300 milligrams) a day does the job. [79]

The good news is that salt has no fat in it. The bad news is that too much salt in your diet can add a number of health problems, including: high blood pressure, increased risk of stroke and heart disease, decreased calcium and subsequent increased risk for osteoporosis, increased risk of stomach cancer. [80]

What's more, each day Americans like you and me take in about twenty to thirty times more salt than our bodies need, without ever adding salt to anything.

How?

Well, salt is included in almost everything you eat, especially packaged foods and restaurant foods. In fact, experts estimate that about 80 percent of your daily salt intake comes from "hidden sources like prepared foods, including fast food." [81] Salt is also in all packaged foods—from frozen dinners to breakfast cereals to canned foods to vegetable drinks to deli meats to soups to sauces to nuts to crackers to condiments to potato chips to pretzels to headache and heartburn medicines to—well, I think you get the idea.

What this means, honestly, is that you never have to add salt to your food in order to get the recommended daily allowance of it. In fact, you're probably already getting too much salt just from your everyday eating anyway. It may be worthwhile for you to simply cut it out of your eating plan, if you can.

Salt is an important ingredient in yeast breads (it's the chemical catalyst that makes the yeast rise in the dough), but in almost all other recipes salt can be cut without affecting the taste or the end result. Additionally, table salt is remarkably unnecessary in your dinner, and can easily be replaced with sodium-free blends such as the Mrs. Dash brand of seasonings.

At my house, we don't add salt to anything, but that's not a hard and fast rule for the *Dude, You Don't Have to be Fat* plan. My recommendation would be that you leave added salt out of your diet and, when possible, buy low-sodium foods. But like sugar and alcohol, this one area where you'll need to decide what's best for your family's lifestyle and buy accordingly.

Okay! That's enough talk about sugar, desserts, alcohol, and salt. Let's move on, and I'll teach you how to become the undisputed King of your kitchen!

Fifteen:
King of the Kitchen!

They say a man's home is his castle.

If that's true, then a man's kitchen is his throne room—the place where his every eating wish is made reality, where policy and pleasure combine to create a thriving kingdom of health and food satisfaction.

From now on, when you step into your kitchen you can be assured that here is where you get to actually live out all the fridge benefits of the three rules we discussed way back on page one of this book:

1. *A man should never be hungry.*
2. *Food is not your enemy*
3. *Eat great. Lose weight. Live well.*

Up to this point, you've learned how to dominate the aisles of your local grocery store. Now, standing in the entrance of your own kitchen, it's time for you to assert your royal manhood over the cabinets and appliances that fill this room. Here's how.

Step 1 for Kitchen Kings: Throw Stuff Out

Listen, Dude, it's time to get serious about your own health. It doesn't do you any good to keep high-fat foods and recipe ingredients in your kitchen where they'll be eaten. So go through your cabinets, your counter tops, and the shelves of your refrigerator and dump anything that doesn't fit the low-fat goals of your new *Dude, You Don't Have to be Fat* lifestyle.

Read the Nutrition Facts labels on the foods you've got, then begin tossing the foods that are high in fat. You need to make room in your kitchen for all the delicious low-fat foods that are going to start filling your home.

Common junk to look for includes: croissants, corn chips, doughnuts, granolas, olives, snack nuts, potato chips, dairy products with fat in them, Crisco and cooking oils, butter and margarine sticks and tubs, fatty red meats, pork, peanut butter, salad dressings with fat in them, mayonnaise with fat in it, fat-filled candies and prepackaged pastries, and pretty much anything that would cause you to eat more than 5 to 8 grams of fat in a single serving for a meal or 2-3 grams of fat in a snack.

If you feel guilty about wasting food that's bad for you, let that remind you not to buy garbage in the first place. Why waste money on food that should be thrown out, and which only harms your body? If you still feel guilty, go ahead and donate your garbage to local food banks (though that has its own moral implications: Why are you giving needy people stuff that's not fit for your own consumption? But we'll let the philosophers debate that issue...). Or give it to wild animals or stuff it in your bird feeder or whatever. The important thing is to kick the fat-heavy freeloaders out of your kitchen.

Next, go ahead and get rid of that deep-fat fryer if you've got one. Believe me, you won't really need, or want, one of those around anymore. (And remind me someday to tell you the story of how, in my misspent youth, I lit my whole kitchen on fire with one of those contraptions.)

If you really-really-really love that deep fat fryer, consider replacing it with an Air-Fryer instead. Air-Fryers aren't perfect, but they do a fine job of using hot air to simulate deep fat frying. I got one last year and it's kind of fun, but after awhile it becomes kind of like that cool toy you got for Christmas, played with for a few weeks, and then forgot about. But still, if you want a deep-fried taste without all that oil, the Air Fryer is a good option for you. You can find them at Walmart, Target, and online.

All right! Now you've got room to load your kitchen with the good stuff.

What this means is that, from now on, anytime you enter your kitchen, you can eat whatever you find there because you know that you've filled it with: a) foods that you like, and b) foods that keep fat intake to a minimum.

It's good to be king, isn't it?

Step 2 for Kitchen Kings:
Use Fat Substitutes

We know that fat (in the form of butter, oil, lard, and many other incarnations) is a common staple in cooking. So what're you supposed to do when that recipe in your cookbook tells you to add a stick of butter or a dozen eggs to your dinner?

Well, first, don't be duped into thinking that every recipe is an ironclad contract. Yeah, I said it. You are the master over what goes into your mouth, and that includes recipe ingredients.

Second, be aware that there are a number of "fat substitutes" you can use when cooking to keep the flavor but banish the fat in your food.

On the pages 92-93 I've given you a list of fat substitutes. These are all substitutes I've used myself and have found both helpful and tasty. Get familiar with this list until you automatically cut-n-paste (cut out fat ingredients, paste in these substitutes) every time you see a new recipe. Or, you know, you can just keep this book in your kitchen and turn to this section whenever you're ready to make a substitute.

Your call, bro. It's your mouth, right?

Step 3 for Kitchen Kings:
Royal Tips for Your New Domain

Now that you've filled your kitchen with tasty, low-fat goodness, and you've learned how to replace the fat in your recipes and cooking projects, you can add on these simple, "extras" below that really multiply your ability to get the most out of a *Dude, You Don't Have to be Fat* kitchen.

What follows for the rest of this chapter are quick-hit summaries of the best advice I've culled from my research and my own experiments in the kitchen. Use them to make your kitchen a lean, mean cooking machine for you and your whole family.

Ready? Here we go...

Be Fat-Substitute Ready.

Always be prepared to use fat substitutes for baking (see notes above). For instance, keep single-serving sizes of applesauce in the cabinet or refrigerator so they're always on hand. Keep an extra block or two of fat-free cream cheese in the fridge. Make sure that when someone in your family is ready to bake, the option of fat substitutes is always readily available.

Be Snack-Ready.

Keep plenty of great-tasting, low-fat or no-fat snacks within easy reach. If you're like most people, whatever is handiest to grab when you're hungry is what goes into your mouth. Make sure fruits and vegetables are the easiest items to grab—and make a rule in your house that sweets are not snacks. Easy snacks could include: fruit, more fruit, low-fat popcorn, pretzels, bagels, turkey pepperoni sticks, low-fat or no-fat crackers, baked chips, thin-sliced deli meat, dry cereals, fruit snacks, low-fat breakfast bars, and so on.

Also, put fruit and veggie snacks in re-sealable, snack-sized plastic bags so they're easy to grab and go. For example, on Sunday night you can prep for the workweek by making a bunch of snack-sized bags of things you like, such as baby carrots or apple slices or orange sections or grapes or sugar snap peas and more. Toss those in your fridge. Then during the week when you're packing your lunch or looking for something quick to eat, you can just grab one of those snack bags and you're good to go.

Braising, Stewing, and Crock-Potting.

When you cook meats in these slow-cooking methods, it actually cooks fat out into the sauce. So before you eat meat you've cooked this way, go ahead and spoon out the liquefied fat and save yourself the trouble of having to digest it later. If you can chill the meat after cooking, the fat will harden and rise to the top, making it even easier to remove.

Butter.

Replace your margarine tubs and butter sticks with fat-free butter spray (such as I Can't Believe It's Not Butter or a generic equivalent). Use this to add buttery flavor to your toast, popcorn, muffins, vegetables, and more—without piling on the fat of margarine or real butter.

Condiments and Sauces.

Keep plenty of fat-free condiments and sauces around, such as ketchup, mustard, Tabasco sauce, salsa, horseradish, Heinz 57 sauce, A-1 sauce, Worcestershire sauce, teriyaki sauce, barbecue sauce, sweet pickle relish, and the like.

Creativity in Your Kitchen!

Invent your own recipes based on foods that are in your low-fat kitchen. Not only will you come up with great meals and snacks that you love—you'll have fun doing it. Invite your kids to join you, and make food creativity a family affair.

Fat Substitutes
for Every Man's Kitchen

Instead of This	Use This Substitute
Any dairy product (cheese, milk, sour cream, whipped cream, half-n-half, cottage cheese, evaporated milk, condensed milk, etc.)	**Fat-free versions of all dairy products.** (Every grocery store should have them.)
Baking chocolate (1 ounce)	**Cocoa powder**. (For every ounce of baking chocolate, use 3 tablespoons of cocoa powder mixed with 2 teaspoons of water instead.)
Butter or margarine in traditional pie crusts.	**A mix of fat-free and light margarine**. (Use about 1/3 of the called-for amount in light margarine, and 2/3 in fat-free margarine)
Butter or margarine spread on breads, pastries, or vegetables	**Fat-free buttery pump sprays** (like I Can't Believe It's Not Butter®)
Eggs	**Egg whites or liquid egg substitute** (For 1 egg, use 2 egg whites and toss the yolks, or use 1/4 cup of Egg Beaters®.)
Mozzarella cheese for pizza topping	**Kraft or Lifetime fat-free mozzarella** or Kraft low-moisture, part-skim mozzarella. (For one large pizza, use 1 3/4 cups of fat-free mozzarella, or 2/3 cup of part-skim. Mix in fat-free cheddar if you like that flavor added.)
Mayonnaise or Miracle Whip	**Fat-free mayonnaise**

Fat Substitutes
for Every Man's Kitchen

Instead of This	Use This Substitute
Oil in cookies, cakes, and brownies	**Applesauce or pureed fruit** (use half the amount of the pureed fruit to replace the oil. For example, if the recipe calls for 1 cup of oil, you'll use 1/2 cup of applesauce. You can also use pureed canned pumpkin in place of the oil. Sounds weird, but tastes good!)
Oil in pancakes, coffee cakes, and sweet breads (such as banana bread or pumpkin bread)	**Fat-free cream cheese, fat-free sour cream, or fat-free plain or vanilla yogurt.** (Use the same amount of any of these as you would oil.)
Oil in sautéed vegetables	**White wine or fat-free chicken broth** (Use about 1/2 cup in the pan, and add liquid as needed while cooking)
Oil or butter for skillet frying	**Non-fat cooking spray** (Pam® or Smart Balance®. You may need to lower the heat a bit when using this spray, and keep a watchful eye so food doesn't burn.)
Traditional pie crust	**Low-fat or no-fat crumbly cookies** (Low-fat gingersnaps, Oreos, graham crackers, or vanilla wafers. Use 1½ cups of cookie crumbs mixed with 3 tablespoons of fat-free vanilla yogurt, and press the mixture into an 8-inch pie plate; spritz with non-fat cooking spray or fat-free butter spray, then bake at 350 degrees for five minutes to set the crust)

Crisco and Oils.

If you haven't done it already, toss out the Crisco. It's entirely fat, and you don't need it. Toss out any other cooking oils hiding in your cabinet as well. If you feel it's necessary, keep one small bottle of olive oil for occasional use, and that's really all you'll need.

Deep-Fried Foods.

Never eat deep-fried foods (that is, food immersed in oil for cooking). That's just eating death boiled in fat. Skillet frying or using an Air-Fryer are both good replacements for deep-fat frying. Also baking with a bread crumb coating is an easy, and tasty, option to replace deep fat frying.

Dressings.

Salad dressings add unnecessary fat to otherwise awesome food. How idiotic is that? When you have salad, if you want dressing use only fat-free varieties (such as fat-free ranch, fat-free Italian, fat-free French, fat-free Catalina, fat-free Thousand Island, and so on). Or try leaving off the dressing and using a splash of red wine vinegar and a dash of black pepper instead. Or spritz fresh lemon juice over your greens.

Most of us don't like our greens dry, so find ways to add a little moisture and flavor that don't add in the fat.

Eggs.

Use egg substitute (such as Egg Beaters or a generic equivalent) for all recipes that require eggs. Typically, 1/4 cup of egg substitute is equal to one egg. Or, as an alternative, use egg whites instead of the whole egg. Remember that two egg whites equal one whole egg.

To separate the yolks from the whites in regular eggs, just crack the egg into your hand and let the white seep through your fingers. Toss the yolk.

Freshen It Up.

Keep fresh foods around as much as possible. Generally the more processed foods are, the more things have been added to them that your body doesn't need. Plus, fresh foods are almost always lower in fat than processed foods, so they're great to keep nearby.

Frozen Dinners.

Keep a full stash of low-fat frozen dinners (such as Lean Cuisine or Healthy Choice or Weight Watchers brands) on hand at all times. When you're hungry for something a little more substantial than a snack, these will be an easy way to fill your stomach without having to think too much about it.

Make sure you check the fat content in specific dinners before you load them in your freezer, though. Most of these meals hit between 3 grams to 7 grams of fat, which is fine—but there are some supposedly "healthy!" recipes that go as high as 12 grams of fat, and they should be avoided.

Frozen Foods.

Frozen fruits and vegetables are handy to keep in your kitchen as you can always add them to a meal or have them for a snack. Frozen fruit blended with fat-free milk or with a fruit juice makes a quick smoothie.

Frying and Baking.

When frying or baking, use a non-fat cooking spray instead of oil or butter on your pan. Use sparingly, though, as a little bit goes a long way.

Mayonnaise.

Never eat mayonnaise with fat—it's just not necessary. Stock your kitchen with fat-free mayonnaise only, and use that as much as you want on sandwiches, salads, and such.

Meats—Cooking.

Grill meat whenever possible. When outdoor grilling is impractical, use a counter-top grilling machine such as the George Foreman Grill. Grilled meat tastes better than most other cooking methods, and also allows fat to liquefy and drip off so you don't have to eat it. Baking meat and then draining fat is also a good option.

Meats—Trimming.

Always cut off visible fat from any cut of meat—even lean ones. If there's a vein of fat marbled into the middle of your meat, fold it in half so that the fat appears on an edge, and trim it out of the center that way. (I saw a Japanese chef do this at a Hibachi restaurant once—it was very cool, and very effective.) Or simply cut your meat into smaller chunks until you can cut out the fatty part.

Pasta and Pizza Sauces.

When cooking or eating pasta or pizza, opt for red sauces with no oil added. These are typically lower in fat, yet taste delicious. Avoid white sauces, which are made with high-fat ingredients like cream and cheese.

Poultry.

Always remove skin from poultry before cooking, and eat only white meat—no dark meat.

Sautéed Foods.

When a recipe calls for something to be sautéed or cooked in oil until tender, you can skip the oil completely. Use white wine or fat-free chicken broth instead to soften those onions, green peppers, mushrooms, or other foods. You can even simmer foods in water, but the flavor is not as good. No matter which liquid you choose, simply pour about a ½ cup into your frying pan, add the vegetables you want sautéed, and cook away. Add more liquid as needed and cook until the food is tender.

Soups.

Always choose broth-based soups instead of cream-based soups. For example, minestrone or chicken noodle are going to be much lower in fat than cream of chicken or broccoli-cheese soup. If you want a cream soup (like cream of mushroom or cream of chicken) always buy the fat-free or low-fat soups made with skim milk. Those work great in casseroles and other recipes. Additionally, soups with tomato base are lower in fat and a good option for you.

Spice it up.

Truth is, taste is one of the top two factors in your eating decisions (price is the other factor), [82] so use your spice cabinet to pump up flavor and eliminate the desire for fat.

Spices are especially tasty in meat and vegetable dishes. A few of my favorites (that you'll always find in my cupboards) are: basil, black pepper, chili powder, cilantro, cinnamon, coriander, cumin, dill, garlic pepper, ginger, lemon pepper, minced garlic, minced onion, mint, nutmeg, oregano, and several of the Mrs. Dash brand of salt-free spice blends. Go ahead and experiment to find out your favorite blends, and use them frequently on your foods.

White Sauces.

Avoid all "white" or cream sauces, such as Alfredo pasta sauce, unless you make them completely fat free with skim milk. Prepackaged versions of these sauces (in prepared meals or stand-alone bottles) are typically made with whole milk and as such are full of unwanted, unnecessary fat.

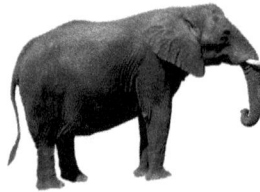

Sixteen:
Eating Fast Food

Charlie Boghosian has made a lot of money off of stupid people.

Perhaps you know him better as Chicken Charlie, the savvy businessman and innovative chef who gave the world such dubious, deep-fried delights as Fried Klondike Bars, Fried Twinkies, Fried Avocados, Fried Girl Scout Cookies, and the heart-stopping Fried Krispy Kreme Chicken Sandwich (two deep-fried doughnuts with a chicken breast wedged between them).

Chicken Charlie sets up his food stand every summer at the San Diego County Fair, and every summer thousands of curious, stupid people fork over cash to see if they can stomach Boghosian's latest fat grenade phenomenon. And business is booming: Recently, in one year alone, Charlie sold more than 100,000 Fried Klondikes. During the past ten years he's also sold more than 2 million Fried Oreo Cookies.

The next item burning up his bestseller list appears to be Fried Kool-Aid— a doughy mixture of flour, water, and Kool-Aid powder that he scoops into little balls and then deep-fries in a hot tub of fat. Two weeks after its summer debut, Charlie had already sold 500 pounds of the fat-sotted Kool-Aid balls.

"It's been huge," he said (without any hint of irony). "People are loving it."

Now, knowing what you do about Chicken Charlie Boghosian, are you surprised to discover that he weighs in at 300+ pounds? That he's a living, breathing example of America's obesity epidemic, both in his physical condition and his fast-food business enterprise? [83] Didn't think so.

Still, the truth is most of us aren't going to make Charlie's Fried Kool-Aid a normal part of our daily diet, so we can grin and shake our heads at his fat-filled, money-hungry antics. But Chicken Charlie does give us a stark visual image of a much larger problem that for just about every American male:

When men eat out, we eat high-fat junk.

Often, we just don't know any better.

At a Glance: Strategies for Fast Food

1) No French fries (or deep-fried anything).
2) No mayonnaise.
3) No dairy (cheese, milk, sour cream, etc.)
4) Be careful about red meats
5) Drink water or juice instead of soda

The Facts

Here are the facts about our ongoing lust affair with fatty fast food and restaurant meals: [84] [85] [86] [87]

• The average American eats about five meals a week away from home. (And this doesn't even include the number of between-meal snacks we also consume!)

• Fast food makes up about three-quarters (75 percent) of all restaurant meals in North America.

• Americans spend in excess of $110 billion dollars on fast food every year.

• Fast food menus are "built on food that's high in fat, high in calories, and dished out in super-large sizes."

• Today about 25 percent of people (one in four) in North America will eat a fast-food meal.

• During the next seven days, the average American adult will eat three hamburgers and four servings of deep-fried French fries at restaurants away from home.

• American families spend nearly half (40 percent) of their food budgets on restaurant meals (both fast-food and sit-down) and other snack foods eaten outside the home.

• Recent studies have shown that "people who eat breakfast or dinner away from home are more likely to be overweight."

• Additional data from the Consumer Reports National Research Center revealed that "the more days per week survey respondents said they ate restaurant or takeout dinners, the greater their weight."

The result of all this eating out? According to Dr. Stephen Sinatra, "Frequent fast-food consumption, with its excessive calories, makes it nearly impossible for the average person to maintain a healthy weight. As a doctor, I see the painful effects of this every single day I go to work." [88]

Now before you assume the worst and decide to drown your sorrows in a super-sized helping of Chicken Charlie's Fried Oreo Cookies, let's bring all this noshing outside the home into perspective. From the *Dude, You Don't Have to be Fat* viewpoint, eating out is not the problem; eating junk is the problem. Let me say that again in a different way that maybe you'll remember:

You're not fat because you eat out, you're fat because you eat junk when you eat out.

Look, it's practically impossible to live in America and not eat restaurant food of some sort. It's even more impossible if you're a corporate professional for whom travel and "business lunches" are the norm. So what are you going to do about it? Cry into your milk-shake? Of course not. You're a *Dude, You Don't Have to be Fat* man. You're smart, you're good-looking, and doggone it, people like you.

Instead of throwing up your hands and surrendering to the Chicken Charlies of this world, you're going to take charge of your eating-out in the same way that you took charge of your kitchen. You're going to eat well—and love it, whether you're at home or away. Here's how.

Remember to Make It Simple & Easy

I love the way *Men's Health* editor, David Zinczenko describes fast-food menu choices that face us whenever we walk through the golden arches. "Trying to decide between two fast-food burgers," he says, "is like deciding which convicted felon you'd ask to house-sit while you're away on vacation." [89]

Yes, it's true that most fast-food restaurants offer limited options, and those options are overwhelming weighted toward high-fat, low-nutrition menu items. That's how they make money—they sell cheap food products, prepared assembly-line fashion, and served by underpaid workers who, honestly, don't give a rip about your weight or health. Still, as

Zinczenko ably points out, "Even if you're making the move through the drive-thru ... you can spare yourself some abdominal agony by making the right food choice." [90]

Now if you're the SMART guy I think you are, you just noticed that I'm suggesting you use the same kind of mindset you used in the grocery store anytime you enter the fast-food restaurant. Perfect! Five gold stars for you, buddy. That's exactly what we're doing.

First, when you go into Burger King or Chipotle or Taco Bell, remember you want to simplify your eating decisions. So as you check out the fast-food menu keep one question in mind: "How much fat is in that?" Choose the lower-fat option every time.

Second, if possible before you go out to eat, plan ahead so you can make it easy to eat well.

"If you're not prepared and you don't have a knowledge base," says certified clinical nutritionist, Kim Bruno, "you're just gonna pick a burger and fries because it's familiar and it's easy." But if you know ahead of time what you like, and what's lower fat on the menu, then you can make an intelligent, and tasty, decision. "You have a little bit more power," says Dr. Bruno, "and then you're not trying to make other people make the same decisions you are." [91]

As far as *Dude, You Don't Have to be Fat* is concerned, Kim Bruno is absolutely on target. Look, I already know that if I'm going to Taco Bell, my best choices are a chicken or steak supreme burrito, fresco style (about 8 grams of fat in either one).

How do I know this?

Well, upon entering the establishment, I attune my spirituality with the netherworld of mother earth until I can literally hear the food ingredients call out to me and say exactly how much fat is contained in each one...

Right. If you believe that, I've got a bridge in San Francisco you might want to buy.

It doesn't take a genius to plan ahead for eating fast food. All I did was hit the Taco Bell website, click on the "Nutrition" link, and skim down the menu until I found lower-fat items listed there. In fact, at Taco Bell I even found a section titled "Drive-Thru Diet® Menu" that lists about a half-dozen menu items with 8 grams of fat or less in each of them. Voila! Good-tasting food with a fat count that's within my daily fat intake goals. Simple as that.

That whole process took me about a minute and a half. You can easily do the same for just about any fast-food restaurant you plan to visit. After a while, you just remember what's good to eat at the restaurants you hit frequently.

Don't have time to access the Internet before you go out to eat fast food? No problem. Ninety-nine percent of these restaurants keep Nutrition Facts info available at the counter for anyone who asks for it. Some places actually put it on a poster somewhere in the restaurant (usually near the counter or close to the bathrooms). Others keep Nutrition Facts brochures on the counter beside the cash register, or at the napkin and condiments counter. A few keep the info in a 3-ring binder behind the counter.

The point is, if you ask, they'll show. So before you order, go ahead and take a minute to ask for a glance at the Nutrition Facts info. Believe me, the world won't end, and no one will look down on you with contempt. Honestly, no one will even care. (Remember, these underpaid high school kids don't give a rat's fuzzy about your health; don't think you're that important to them, okay?)

However, if you find yourself eating out without having had the opportunity to plan ahead, then fall back on your simplified plan for eating decisions:

Low-Fat or No-Fat = Good Eats.
NOT Low-Fat or No-Fat = Crap.

Here are five quick ways to lower your fat intake at pretty much any fast-food restaurant in America:

1) No French fries (or "fried" anything).
You know that anything cooked by frying in hot oil is literally soaked in, and dripping with, fat. Just say no, bro. Diarrhea and weight gain are not pleasant follow-ups to a fast-food meal anyway. So leave the French fries for the fatties in your group.

Also avoid any chicken sandwich that's coated with batter and deep-fried. Skip anything that's advertised as "chicken-fried" or "crisped" or even just "fried." Those are all cooked in a vat of fat. Opt for grilled sandwiches instead, and fruit or low-fat yogurt choices as a side. Just about every single hamburger joint has some version of a "grilled chicken sandwich" as an option, so make that your fall-back choice if you don't know how much fat is in other menu items.

2) No mayonnaise--ever.
Speaking of a grilled chicken sandwich, if you go to Burger King and order a delicious TenderGrill Chicken Sandwich on Ciabatta bread, the default protocol is to slap about 1 tablespoon of mayonnaise on the bun. That's kind of like dipping your food in a toilet before eating it.

With mayonnaise, this otherwise healthy, delicious sandwich racks up 18 grams of fat. If you add three words when ordering, "Hold the mayo," you knock 11 grams of fat out of that sandwich, making it a tasty choice with only 7 grams of fat total.

So always—always—say "hold the mayo" when you order fast food.

3) No dairy (cheese, milk, sour cream, etc.).
The other common ingredient on just about any fast-food menu item, from burgers to burritos to grilled chicken sandwiches and more, is cheese. Trouble is, America's fast-food royalty are stubborn-stupid, insisting on using dairy products made with whole milk instead of skim milk in their foods. That means whenever you allow a fast-food worker to add a slice of cheese on your sandwich, or to sprinkle shredded cheese on your salad, or to add sour cream to your burrito, you are literally letting that person smear unnecessary fat all over your food.

For instance, a single, flimsy, near-tasteless slice of American cheese on your Tender-Grill Chicken Sandwich adds 3 full grams to your fat total—nearly half the amount of the rest of the sandwich as a whole. Worth it? Nope.

So, as you get into the habit of saying, "Hold the mayo," go ahead and also learn to say, "No cheese or dairy products." (That'll also help you avoid trouble from places that grill their buns with butter pasted on.)

4) Be careful about red meats.
Not all red meats are high in fat, but most are.

For instance, a Carl's Junior Original Six Dollar Burger packs on 54 grams of fat in a single serving. That's because fast-food burger-makers tend to use lower quality beef or ground chuck for your hamburger—the cheap stuff you'd find in your grocery store with 30 percent fat content or at best 20 percent fat (a whopping 21 grams of fat per serving). You definitely don't need that junk in your system, bro.

Compare that to the Carl's Junior Charbroiled Barbecue Chicken sandwich: only 7 grams of fat, and you can see what a difference a meat makes.

So in almost all cases, hamburgers are going to be a bad choice for your *Dude, You Don't Have to be Fat* lifestyle. The rare, and welcome, exception is occasionally steak in a fast-food sandwich or burrito. Because steak menu items are considered more "prestige," they're often trimmed of fat and can be almost as lean as chicken. This is true in Taco Bell burritos, as well as in Qdoba and Chipotle burritos.

One word of warning, though: If you don't know ahead of time that your fast-food place is using lean meat for steak, don't order it. Especially in steak sandwiches that can be a bad idea, because often steak sandwiches are basted with butter (even more pure fat!) before being cooked.

So, generally speaking, grilled chicken will always be a safer bet for you. But don't be afraid to check Nutrition Facts on steak menu items—you may be pleasantly surprised.

5) Drink water or juice instead of soda.

Honestly, there's no fat in the sodas served at your fast-food restaurant, so if you feel good about your eating choices there it's probably no big deal to order a Dr Pepper with your lunch. At the same time, fast-food choices are often heavier in fat overall than what you'd eat at home, so I'd recommend that you go ahead and cut the sugar consumption that comes with a soda order when eating out. After all, you never drink just one over-sized cup of the stuff, which makes it easier to overdo it on your sugar intake—and we know that can easily be transformed into fat within your body.

I typically drink water at a fast-food place; saves me money, and it keeps me from the possibility of taking in too much fat-inducing sugar.

Follow those five precautions faithfully when eating at a fast-food place, and you should do just fine—and can enjoy the camaraderie and friendship that goes along with a quick lunch out with your coworkers.

Now, what about when you eat at a sit-down restaurant?

Well, here's what you can do...

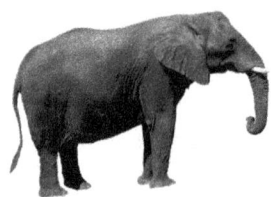

Seventeen:
Fine Dining

Just as we do at the grocery store and at fast-food restaurants, we're going to simplify our eating decisions when working through a sit-down restaurant menu.

Remember:

> Low-Fat or No-Fat = Good Eats.
> NOT Low-Fat or No-Fat = Crap.

Truth is, the way food is prepared has as much to do with its fat content as the original amount of fat contained in the food itself—and restaurants are notorious for adding unneeded, and unwanted fat, to otherwise healthy food.

Consider:

An onion has only trace amounts of fat in it ... until Outback Steakhouse turns it into a Bloomin' Onion. Once they're done battering it up, death-frying it, and serving it on a plate for you, it's got 82 artery-clogging grams of fat.

So to paraphrase Jerry McGuire, you've got to help the restaurant help you. Here are five ways to lower your fat intake at when you go out for a meal at a fine dining establishment:

1) Look for the Right Code Words

Yes, you know what the word "fried" means on a menu, but what about all those other crazy cooking terms you find there? Ever thought you were ordering something low-fat only to see it served on a plate covered with cheese sauce or sour cream or drenched in butter? That's happened to me many times, until my wife finally took pity on me and started explaining the secret cooking codes used in most restaurants.

If you understand the terms commonly used on menus or in naming of dishes, you can get a handle on what's going to show up on your plate. That kind of knowledge can make a world of difference in the way you order—and what you actually eat.

And don't worry, you don't have to memorize and then try to translate all the fine dining lingo. You can use the chart starting on page 125 to help you decipher it all.

At a Glance: Strategies for Fine Dining

1) Look for the Right Code Words
2) No fried foods
3) Lie about dairy allergies
4) Sauces and Condiments ALWAYS on the side
5) Drink Juices or Teas instead of Soda

2) No fried foods

This should go without saying, but because deep-fried foods are so much a part of America's dining experience, I want to emphasize it again for you here.

Hey Dude—if it says "fried" on the menu, stay away from it. It's full of fat added in during cooking process and is not worth your time and appetite. You can do better, bro.

3) Lie about dairy allergies

Ancient philosophers reasoned that there were four circumstances in which it was ethical to lie:

1) To save a life;
2) To save a friendship;
3) To mislead and enemy;
4) To maintain peace in the home.

For you, just because you're special, I'm going add a fifth circumstance in which it's okay for you to lie:

5) *When ordering a meal at a restaurant.*

Every time you order food at a restaurant, tell your server this white lie: "Will you please inform the chef that I'm allergic to dairy, and to prepare my food accordingly?"

Now, I thought I was the only one who did this, but it turns out this is actually a strategy recommended by some dietitians as well. [92] So, you know, take that everybody who said I was nuts to lie about having a dairy allergy.

Here's the thing: You have to remember that even in a fancy, upscale restaurant, food is still an assembly-line business. Your server may smile at you and act like you are the only customer the kitchen is worried about ... but look around you:

Everybody in the place wants food. And they all want it now.

Meanwhile, back in the kitchen...

A chef is cooking up six portions of this and a dozen side orders of that—all in a row, all uniform in content, and often pre-cooked or pre-mixed to some extent—all of which can easily be transferred to a plate and taken to your table.

Then you enter and try to tell your waitress what seems to be a complicated, interruptive request like:

"Please, no cheese on this item, and leave the sour cream off of that one, and please no butter on my bread rolls or side potato and..."

Sure, your waitress is smiling and nodding, but in her head she's thinking, "What a hassle; this guy will never notice if there's a little butter on his bread or if that sauce has sour cream in it..."

Right away you've got only a 50/50 chance of getting what you've ordered. (Trust me, I speak from experience.) If your requests do make it back to the chef, you're still one of a dozen standardized plates he or she is creating. Again, you've only got about a 50/50 chance of getting what you need. So listen to me on this:

One of the easiest ways to eliminate large amounts of fat in a restaurant meal is simply to remove the high-fat dairy products that chefs like to use in their recipes: cheese, cream sauces and dressings, sour cream, butter, buttermilk, and so on. So instead of the long litany above, just tell your server this:

"Will you please inform the chef that I'm allergic to dairy, and to prepare my food accordingly?"

You know what your server—and the chef—are thinking then?

"Lawsuit warning! Better make sure there's no cheese, sour cream, butter, etc. in this guy's meal, and we probably should cook it in a freshly cleaned pan so no butter residue from a previous meal gets in his food. Otherwise, if this guy has an allergic reaction, we could get sued."

Guess what?

When your plate comes, there'll be no high-fat dairy products on it anywhere. Since I started lying about dairy allergies, I've had a 99 percent success rate in eliminating those fatty ingredients when eating out. So make it easy on everybody next time; just tell a white lie about dairy and enjoy your dinner—without all the fat.

4) Sauces and Condiments ALWAYS on the side

Many unwanted fats and oils are in the sauces and dressings poured over foods, and these can be easily avoided or only sparingly used. Still, it's often hard to tell from a menu if a sauce or condiment has been made with oil or cream as an ingredient—and sometimes (well, often) your server will have no idea what's in the gunk he's delivering to you.

So if a food comes with sauces or condiments, or if it appears that an unwanted item is added to your food at the end of the cooking process—such as a sauce or a heavy covering of cheese—tell the server, "On the side, please." Then you can check out the sauce or condiment and decide for yourself if it's okay to spread all over your food.

5) Drink Juices or Teas instead of Soda or Alcohol

Yes, it's true that soda and alcohol typically don't have fat in them, so in that sense they can be a part of your *Dude, You Don't Have to be Fat* eating plan. HOWEVER, we also know that sugared sodas and most alcoholic beverages don't offer any real nutrients for your system, and that they can easily be stored as fat cells within your body. Plus, drinking one soda or alcoholic drink almost always leads to drinking more than one of those things as your meal progresses.

I'd suggest that you just avoid them both when you eat out. Try flavored (but not sugared) teas or fruit juices instead. Or even better, just drink water with a lemon slice in it. That's the most refreshing, nutritious, and thirst-quenching beverage of all drinks offered—and it's free.

All right! You're ready to eat out with the best of them! So go ahead and plan an elegant date with your favorite girl, and enjoy.

"Ah Mikey," you say, "that's all well and good, but what do I do when I'm invited to a friend's house for dinner, or going to a party where food will be served? What then?"

Read on, my brother. Read on...

Cheat Sheet:
Restaurant Code Words
(part one)

Code Word	What It Means	Advice
Alfredo	Cheese & cream-based sauce	Avoid
Au Gratin	Food covered with cheese or bread crumbs and butter	Avoid
Au Jus	The drippings or juice from the meat. Usually no fat is added (although it may contain some fat from the meat); used as an alternative to gravy	Enjoy!
Baked	Oven-Cooked using dry heat	Enjoy! But instruct your server not to use any butter or dairy, or oil-based marinade on your baked food
Blanched	The food has been dropped into boiling water, then quickly plunged into cold water. It's a fast way of cooking that keeps foods (typically vegetables) crunchy and can remove unwanted peelings as well	Enjoy!
Braised	Slowly cooked in a tightly covered pan	Enjoy! But ask your server to remove any excess fat separated out by the braising process
Broiled	Cooked under an overhead heat source	Enjoy! But instruct your server not to use any butter or dairy or oil-based marinade on your baked food
Buttery	Hey Dude, this doesn't mean it just tastes like butter. It means there really is butter in it!	Avoid
Creamed (also, Creamy, or In Cream Sauce)	Cream and butter are added to your food	Avoid
Crisped	Fried in oil	Avoid

Cheat Sheet:
Restaurant Code Words
(part two)

Code Word	What It Means	Advice
Fried (also, Pan-Fried, Oven-Fried, Lightly-Fried, etc.)	Fried in oil	Avoid
Grilled	Cooked over an open flame (this allows some fat to liquefy and drip off your food).	Enjoy! but instruct your server not to use any butter or dairy or oil-based marinade on your grilled food
Hollandaise Sauce (or any sauce that ends in "aise")	Your food is covered in a sauce made mostly of egg yolks and butter	Avoid
Loaded	High-fat ingredients have been added to your food (such as butter, bacon, sour cream, cheese, and so on).	Avoid
Poached	Your food is boiled, steamed, or simmered in water	Enjoy!
Roasted	Usually means baked, but marinades, oils, or cream-based gravies may have been poured over during the cooking process	Enjoy! But instruct your server not to use any butter or dairy, or oil-based marinade, or added gravies on your roasted food
Sautéed	Cooked in butter or oil	Avoid
Steamed	Cooked over (but not in) boiling water; a particularly flavorful way to prepare rice and other vegetables, along with some meats	Enjoy!
Tender	Usually refers to meat with high fat content	Avoid

As you can see, even if a food is prepared in a desirable manner, the restaurant can thwart your good intentions by adding butter or dairy or oil to your food!

I've been disappointed more than once to find my steamed broccoli had been covered with butter before being brought to my table. I've learned it's very important to talk to your server and ask for further clarification before ordering. Even if you've figured out how to skip sautéed vegetables and choose grilled ones instead, if a spoonful of oil is ladled over the top, you're good plans just went out the window. Eater Beware!

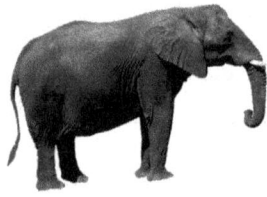

Eighteen:
Eating Socially

When my son was in kindergarten, he attended a birthday party for a friend of his from school. Like all five-year-olds, he played hard, ate lots of sugar, and generally had a great time. In fact, he had so much fun that he wanted to share it.

For some reason, when Tony was little, he thought wearing snow boots in summertime was pretty much the coolest thing in the world. So he wore them everywhere—including to his friend's birthday party.

Imagine the, um, joy (?) my wife felt when Tony came home and proudly announced to her, "I saved you a treat from the party!" Then he reached INSIDE his sweaty, dirty, sticky snow boot and pulled out a mangled Gummy Worm he'd brought home especially for her.

What could Amy do?

There was her cherubic, thoughtful little boy offering her a truly disgusting candy treat! She did what any of us would do:

She ate it.

Tony bounced away happily; Amy felt sick, but it was worth it to protect the self-esteem of that precious little boy.

Now, when it comes to eating at friends' houses or noshing on snacks at a party, some guys feel like they have the same obligation to their hosts that Amy had to our son. "Hey, if they serve it, I should it eat," they say. Well, here's the truth:

Those guys are idiots. Don't be one of them.

Yes, if your delightful preschooler "cooks" up a treat for you, sure, go ahead and swallow enough of the garbage to safeguard her self-esteem. That's just part of what it means to be a dad. But don't confuse your angel-faced child with your buddies from work or church or from around the neighborhood. In case you didn't get this when you turned 18, rules are different for adults than they are for kids. It's your body and you have the right to choose healthful foods for it—adults already understand that.

Think about it.

If you're a non-smoker and you go to your friend's house, do you have any problem declining the offer of a cigarette? Is your buddy hurt and offended that you opted not to suck cancer-causing smoke into your lungs like he does? Of course not. He

Strategies for Eating at a Friends' or at Parties

1) Talk to your friends.
2) Offer to bring food to the meal.
3) Suggest an alternative
4) Don't go hungry to a party.
5) Look for the lighter side of party foods.

understands that physical health is a matter of personal choice. He chooses to risk cancer for the thrill of nicotine; you choose not to.

Yet when that same friend puts a slice of chocolate-pecan pie in front of you, you feel obligated to eat every last crumb, even though you know it's laden with fat and can lead to all kinds of diseases including heart attacks, stroke, diabetes, and more. And your lame excuse is, "I don't want to offend my friend."

Puh-lease. You're a man, not a wimp who has no control over his own mouth.

If your friend served you some food you find disgusting like, say liver or pinto bean pie, my guess is you wouldn't worry too much about your friend's feelings before politely declining to eat that stuff. And your friend wouldn't be offended if you told him, "You know, I don't really like pinto beans in a pie, but thanks anyway."

And besides, we're talking about your friend. This person likes you already; he'll understand. He'll probably support you. He may even join you.

I remember once our family was spending a day with friends. (Let's give them fake names to preserve their privacy: Mick and Helen.) When it came time for dinner, Helen started cooking up food in the kitchen while we "helped" (meaning, basically, we hung around and chatted while she did all the work ... sorry Helen!). First she made burgers and fries for all the kids. Mick turned toward me sympathetically and said, "Wow, too bad you can't eat this Mike. It smells delicious. What a shame for you, huh?" I didn't actually call Mick a moron, but I did tell him I knew what was coming for me, and I wasn't disappointed at all by it.

Next Helen started cooking for the adults. Because she knew I was a *Dude, You Don't Have to be Fat* kind of guy, she'd planned to make seasoned, grilled chicken for me, along with steamed broccoli and a big hunk of warm French bread. Because Helen isn't stupid, she also went ahead and made enough of the chicken and broccoli for her as well, and then she started grilling Mick's burger. When Mick saw my plate, sizzling with juicy chicken breast and more, his mouth dropped open. The dinner Helen prepared for me looked (and tasted!) like it had been made at a fine-dining restaurant.

"Wait a minute," Mick said, "I want that instead of a lousy hamburger!" Too bad for him, he was stuck with his fat-filled greaseburger and chubby fries. An hour later he was bloated and gassy and uncomfortable. I was full and satisfied.

Guess what happened next time we ate over at Mick and Helen's? Yep, we all had the tasty, lower-fat options—even the kids. And we all enjoyed every bite.

So, my point is, you're not doing anybody any favors by abandoning the benefits of healthy eating in your life when you go to a friend's place for dinner ... but you might do everybody a favor by sharing your lifestyle with those closest to you. Food for thought.

Meanwhile, let's talk about five healthy tactics you can employ next time you're invited to eat at a friend's home or at a party.

1) Talk to Your Friends

You know what I do when somebody invites me over for a meal? I say, "I'd love to come over, but I want you to know that I have some unique eating habits. Will that be a problem?"

Want to know how many times my friends have said, "Yes, that's a problem. You'll have to just eat whatever we serve." *Zero.*

Hey, they're friends inviting you into a social setting. As hosts, they want you to be comfortable, and they're often grateful when you communicate your needs to them instead of keeping that kind of information secret.

And just to be clear, I've said that same line to close friends, to brand-new friends, to work friends, even to the president of the book company where my wife works. And let me point out again: Not a single person has ever been offended or angry with me for informing them that I need to eat lower-fat foods. Not one.

Now, they may need to be educated a bit on what kinds of foods and cooking techniques yield lower fat counts, but when people invite you over they are already motivated to be accommodating. Give your friends a chance, and don't assume the worst about them. I think you'll be happy with the way they respond.

2) Offer to Bring Food to the Meal

Seriously, were you raised in a barn or something? It's just common courtesy to offer to bring some part of the meal when you're invited to a friend's home for dinner. So be a gentleman and offer to bring food along on your visit.

For starters, if your friend seems to be having trouble understanding how to prepare a lower-fat entrée, you can offer to bring your own main dish. Just tell a white lie and say, "I'm on a special diet, so would it be okay if I brought my own main dish?" (Right, I know, *Dude, You Don't Have to be Fat* not a diet, it's a lifestyle, but it takes too long to explain that to others so just use the "diet" word and don't worry about it.) Very few hosts or hostesses are going to give you a problem about that.

If your host or hostess seems to have the main dish thing covered, then you bring a couple of side dishes, such as bread and a fruit salad, or a side dish and dessert, like a low-fat broccoli casserole and sweet lemonade pie (see page 204). The idea here is simple: Bring stuff you know you can eat. They'll think you're a generous, well-mannered person; you'll be assured that there's something you can eat at the table.

This also helps protect you against misunderstanding. For instance, we once went to dinner at a friend's home, and were pleased when our gracious hostess gladly set fresh, steamed vegetables and rice on the table—then horrified when she proceeded to pour butter and cheese on top of it all. If you bring your own sides or desserts, you can avoid letting your hostess make that kind of social blunder with your meal.

3) Suggest an Alternative

This option is not always ideal, but if you've been to a friend's house once for dinner and found that they simply were unable to deliver reasonably low-fat options for you, then try suggesting an alternative the next time you want to get together.

For instance, if you're invited over for a meal, but you're unsure that you can get the kinds of food your new *Dude, You Don't Have to be Fat* body wants and needs, then offer to turn the tables. Say in effect, "Hey, we should get together—that sounds fun! But because I have special needs when it comes to eating, how about if we have dinner at my house this time?" Voila—you've just accepted a dinner invitation, and also generously given one as well. You win both ways. Let your friend bring along whatever food he and his family want to add to the meal, and enjoy yourselves.

You can also redirect the invitation so that it doesn't involve a meal. Remember, eating together is actually a social activity, a means to spend time with a friend, but there are other ways to spend time together that don't revolve around a meal.

Ask your friend to join you for a round of golf instead of brunch. Suggest that you hang out at a sporting event or an art gallery. Go on an adventure to find the coolest Classic Arcade Games place in your area. Put your creative mind to use and think of other things you can do with friends that don't mean you'll need to eat together.

4) Don't Go To a Party with an Empty Stomach

Eating with friends at a party is a bit different than going to someone's house for a meal, simply because of the number of people involved. When your host is preparing food for just you and your family, it's fairly easy to accommodate your food health needs. However, when a host is preparing snacks for a large group of people, necessity requires that he or she simply buy and prepare foods in bulk. In these situations, you just have to assume you won't find much that's worthwhile to eat at the party. So we come to the obvious solution:

Don't be hungry when there's nothing worthwhile to eat nearby.

Remember the "M" in the fight SMART strategies? Make it *easy* to eat well.

If you go to a party on an empty stomach, you're just asking for trouble. So eat ahead of time, just before you go to the shindig. If you get there and there's good stuff after all, you can snack lightly anyway. But (more likely) if you get there and it's all frozen, fried foods and garbage, you can simply skip the food table and have fun hanging out with your friends without stuffing junk down your throat. Either way, you win.

I usually eat a sandwich, or a small bowl of leftovers, or a heavy snack before I go to a get-together. That way I'm not hungry when I get there—but I'm not too stuffed to snack on something if the food turns out to be good. For longer parties (such as Super Bowl parties or New Year's Eve parties) I also bring along food I can eat as the night wears on. Most hosts don't mind if you stash a sub sandwich in their refrigerator during the party, or you can also bring along foods that don't need to be refrigerated (like crackers and fruit slices) and keep them within easy reach in your car for when you get hungry.

5) Look for the Lighter Side of Party Foods

While you can't count on there being anything worthwhile to eat at a party, you can always see what's available and find the lower-fat gems among the heart-stopping fried cheese sticks and chocolate cheesecake truffles. A few lower-fat options that you might find are:

- bread chunks (choose dry sourdough or dry wheat, if possible)
- deli lunch meats (choose thin-sliced chicken, turkey, or roast beef)
- fruit platters (always delicious)
- hummus dip (yes, this does have a little olive oil in it, but if you lightly dip veggies or bread chunks in it, you should be fine)
- Italian ice desserts (tasty, sweet, and only trace amounts of fat!)
- shrimp cocktail (surprisingly low fat, and many people like the taste)
- vegetable platters

If you find any of these lower-fat items on the food tables at your next party, you're all set. Just fill up on those things while everyone else chugs the flubber items.

And hey, have a good time, Dude!

Nineteen:
And Now...

My son, you are now a man.
A Dude, You Don't Have to be Fat *man, to be exact.*

Congratulations! You've now got everything you need to live a life filled with all the "fridge benefits" you can muster. Let's face it … you're one very cool guy. You're well on your way to achieving all your food health dreams and goals.

From now on you are going to:

- Take charge of your own body—and see the difference in your mirror.
- Demand "fridge benefits" anyplace you eat—at home, at a restaurant, at a fast-food place, or even at a friend's house for dinner.
- Live out a simple approach to eating well—and loving it.
- Enjoy your food—without letting it harm you.
- Feel better about yourself, your body, your life, and your future.
- Make your refrigerator an ally instead of your enemy.
- Get off the fad diet and get-skinny-quick treadmills.
- Become smarter, healthier, and more confident.
- Love your lifestyle—and live longer to boot.

Before I skip out, I want to do a few last things for you. First, I want to encourage you to take a good look at the "Mini-Cookbook for Men" I've included at the end of this book. These are all kitchen-tested, guy-friendly recipes you're going to love.

Use theses recipes to eat well (and love it!)—and to impress your friends and family members with your culinary skills. You don't even have to tell them that everything in there is low fat—they won't even notice. Just enjoy the food, enjoy the health it provides, and enjoy being a kitchen stud and all that goes along with that.

Next, I want you to notice that, in the section immediately following this chapter, I've included a bunch of charts and tables and random info for you.

If there was a chart you saw earlier in the book, you can find it quickly and easily in this section instead of having to dig back through the chapters in hopes of finding that specific info again.

Also, there are extra charts and bonus info in that section (like "Best Choices for Fast Food") that you may want to check out from time to time. I put this stuff in this book cuz I thought you might want it, so feel free to come back to it anytime.

Last, but not least, I want to remind you one more time of the three rules of a *Dude, You Don't Have to be Fat* lifestyle:

1. *A man should never be hungry.*
2. *Food is not your enemy*
3. *Eat great. Lose weight. Live well.*

Those rules govern everything about the *Dude, You Don't Have to be Fat* plan. Let them guide you each day as you live out your new food health.

Now, it's time for you to live the rest of your life—and love it.

Enjoy!

Mike Nappa

Part 4

Charts, References, & Other Helpful Info

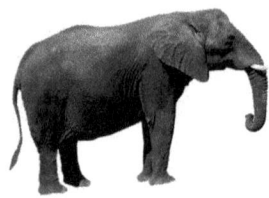

Weight Chart A:
Ideal Weights for Men
(estimated) [93]

Height	Ideal Weight*		
	Smaller Build	Medium Build	Large Build
5' 2"	128-134 pounds	131-141 pounds	138-150 pounds
5' 3"	130-136 pounds	133-143 pounds	140-153 pounds
5' 4"	132-138 pounds	135-145 pounds	142-156 pounds
5' 5"	134-140 pounds	137-148 pounds	144-160 pounds
5' 6"	136-142 pounds	139-151 pounds	146-164 pounds
5' 7"	138-145 pounds	142-154 pounds	149-168 pounds
5' 8"	140-148 pounds	145-157 pounds	152-172 pounds
5' 9"	142-151 pounds	148-160 pounds	155-176 pounds
5' 10"	144-154 pounds	151-163 pounds	158-180 pounds
5' 11"	146-157 pounds	154-166 pounds	161-184 pounds
6' 0"	149-160 pounds	157-170 pounds	164-188 pounds
6' 1"	152-164 pounds	160-174 pounds	168-192 pounds
6' 2"	155-168 pounds	164-178 pounds	172-197 pounds
6' 3"	158-172 pounds	167-182 pounds	176-202 pounds
6'4"	162-176 pounds	171-187 pounds	181-207 pounds

*Note: Be aware that "Ideal Weight" is a target, not necessarily your exact weight requirement. I've found that most men who get within 5-10 pounds of their ideal weight do very well in terms of health, well-being, and appearance.

Weight Chart B:
Recommended Fat Intake Per Day
by Target Weight*

(Assuming 10 percent of daily calories from fat)

Target Weight	Recommended Fat Intake Per Day
125 pounds	21 grams
130 pounds	22 grams
135 pounds	23 grams
140 pounds	23 grams
145 pounds	24 grams
150 pounds	25 grams
155 pounds	26 grams
160 pounds	27 grams
165 pounds	28 grams
170 pounds	28 grams
175 pounds	29 grams
180 pounds	30 grams
185 pounds	31 grams
190 pounds	32 grams
195 pounds	33 grams
200 pounds	33 grams

***Note**: For other target weights (assuming 10 percent of daily calories from fat), use this mathematical formula and round to the nearest whole number:

Target Weight × 0.1667 = Recommended Fat Intake Per Day, in Grams

Dude, You Don't Have to be Fat

USDA "MyPlate"

Based on the USDA 2010 Dietary Guidelines for Americans, the MyPlate graphic is designed to help you get a clear visual image of what a healthy meal should look like. A few notes:

• **A typical healthy meal includes all five food groups**: Fruit, vegetables, grains, proteins, and dairy. (For more on these groups, see chapters ten – thirteen of *Dude, You Don't Have to be Fat*).
• **Fill half your plate with fruits and vegetables**. Fruit and vegetables offer the best nutrients for your body, so eat a lot, and eat 'em often.
• **Keep protein servings at less than 25 percent of your plate** (typically about 5 ounces a day). Think of meat as a side dish rather than a main dish, and always opt for "extra lean" cuts.
• **For grains shoot for about 25 percent - 30 percent of your plate**. (This is food such as breads, rolls, rice, cereals, and the like) More importantly, make sure your grain-based foods include plenty of whole grains. USDA suggests a minimum of half the grains on your plate be whole grains.
• **For dairy, USDA suggests about 1 cup per meal**, which could be in a glass of milk, or in cheese in an entree, or in yogurt or any other dairy variation on your plate. always make this serving fat-free (or "skim") to glean all the best benefits of milk—without any of the harmful side effects of fat.
• **For more information, visit ChooseMyPlate.gov**

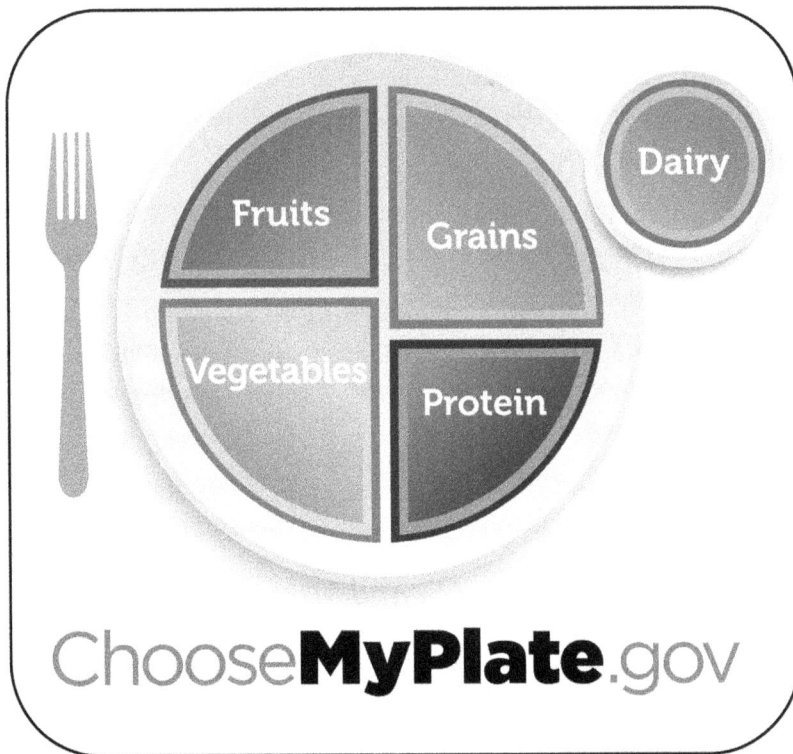

How to Read a Nutrition Facts Label

A. Serving Size

Check here first to see how the manufacturer defines a "serving" of this food. Be aware that some food producers try to shrink the serving size in order to give the appearance of a lower-fat product—so judge the serving size based on what you will actually eat. For instance, a serving size of "four ounces" for meat is about average and should be accurate. A serving size of "five chips" is ridiculously low (most people eat between 15-20 potato chips in a serving), and so you'd want to multiply all numbers below by three or four to reflect your realistic serving size.

B. Calories

This line will tell you the total number of calories in each serving, as well as what percentage of those calories are derived from fat. This can be helpful if you're counting daily calories along with daily fat intake. Otherwise, it's mostly just FYI for you.

C. % Daily Value

This column simply tells you how each item relates to the USDA's recommended daily allowances. It can be helpful as a general guideline, but because it's based only on a 2000 calorie diet and ignores a wide number of variables (such as the fact that the USDA recommends about three times more fat than you actually need), it's not entirely reliable for your *Dude, You Don't Have to be Fat* plan. Feel free to ignore it.

D. Total Fat

For your purposes as a *Dude, You Don't Have to be Fat* man, this is the most important line on the whole Nutrition Facts label. It tells you exactly how many grams of fat are in a serving, and thus it tells you how many fat grams you'll be "spending" from your daily allowance of fat grams (see Weight Chart B, page 118) when you eat this product. Get used to always checking this line on the Nutrition Facts label.

E. Cholesterol and Sodium

These two lines will tell you how much cholesterol and sodium are in a serving of this food. Typically, the lower the numbers here, the better for you.

F. Total Carbohydrates

Here you'll find information about how much fiber and sugars are included in a serving. Typically, higher fiber and lower amounts of sugar are desired.

G. Protein

This tells you how many grams of protein are in each serving of your food. Since *Dude, You Don't Have to be Fat* doesn't typically track protein grams, this info is mostly FYI for you.

H. Vitamins and Minerals

Here you'll get a glimpse of all the vitamins and minerals found in the food, listed as a percentage of the USDA's daily recommendations. Typically, you want to see higher numbers here, as that means you are getting more of the nutrients that help your body thrive.

I. Footnotes

This section is just a standard summary of USDA recommendations and other basic information. Feel free to ignore it, unless you need a refresher.

Nutrition Facts

4 servings per container

(A) → **Serving size**   **3/4 cup**

Amount Per Serving

(B) → **Calories**   **150**

% Daily Value* ← (C)

(D) → **Total Fat** 1g	**1%**
Saturated Fat 0g	**0%**
Trans Fat 0g	
(E) → **Cholesterol** 255mg	**85%**
Sodium 300mg	**13%**
(F) → **Total Carbohydrate** 400g	**145%**
Dietary Fiber 4g	**14%**
Total Sugars 8g	
Includes 0g Added Sugars	**0%**
(G) → **Protein** 2g	**4%**

Not a significant source of vitamin D, calcium, iron, and potassium ← (H)

* The % Daily Value (DV) tells you how much a nutrient in a serving of food contributes to a daily diet. 2,000 calories a day is used for general nutrition advice. ← (I)

Fat Substitutes
for Every Man's Kitchen

Instead of This	Use This Substitute
Any dairy product (cheese, milk, sour cream, whipped cream, half-n-half, cottage cheese, evaporated milk, condensed milk, etc.)	**Fat-free versions of all dairy products.** (Every grocery store should have them.)
Baking chocolate (1 ounce)	**Cocoa powder.** (For every ounce of baking chocolate, use 3 tablespoons of cocoa powder mixed with 2 teaspoons of water instead.)
Butter or margarine in traditional pie crusts.	**A mix of fat-free and light margarine.** (Use about 1/3 of the called-for amount in light margarine, and 2/3 in fat-free margarine)
Butter or margarine spread on breads, pastries, or vegetables	**Fat-free buttery pump sprays** (like I Can't Believe It's Not Butter®)
Eggs	**Egg whites or liquid egg substitute** (For 1 egg, use 2 egg whites and toss the yolks, or use 1/4 cup of Egg Beaters®.)
Mozzarella cheese for pizza topping	**Kraft or Lifetime fat-free mozzarella** or Kraft low-moisture, part-skim mozzarella. (For one large pizza, use 1 3/4 cups of fat-free mozzarella, or 2/3 cup of part-skim. Mix in fat-free cheddar if you like that flavor added.)
Mayonnaise or Miracle Whip	**Fat-free mayonnaise**

Fat Substitutes
for Every Man's Kitchen

Instead of This	Use This Substitute
Oil in cookies, cakes, and brownies	**Applesauce or pureed fruit** (use half the amount of the pureed fruit to replace the oil. For example, if the recipe calls for 1 cup of oil, you'll use 1/2 cup of applesauce. You can also use pureed canned pumpkin in place of the oil. Sounds weird, but tastes good!)
Oil in pancakes, coffee cakes, and sweet breads (such as banana bread or pumpkin bread)	**Fat-free cream cheese, fat-free sour cream, or fat-free plain or vanilla yogurt.** (Use the same amount of any of these as you would oil.)
Oil in sautéed vegetables	**White wine or fat-free chicken broth** (Use about 1/2 cup in the pan, and add liquid as needed while cooking)
Oil or butter for skillet frying	**Non-fat cooking spray** (Pam® or Smart Balance®. You may need to lower the heat a bit when using this spray, and keep a watchful eye so food doesn't burn.)
Traditional pie crust	**Low-fat or no-fat crumbly cookies** (Low-fat gingersnaps, Oreos, graham crackers, or vanilla wafers. Use 1½ cups of cookie crumbs mixed with 3 tablespoons of fat-free vanilla yogurt, and press the mixture into an 8-inch pie plate; spritz with non-fat cooking spray or fat-free butter spray, then bake at 350 degrees for five minutes to set the crust)

Cheat Sheet:
Advertising Code Words

Code Word	What it Means	Advice
Fat-Free	Less than 0.5 (one-half) gram of fat per serving.	It is strange that something "Fat-Free" could actually contain up to one-half gram of fat ... but that's not usually a big deal. Enjoy "Fat-Free" as much as you want.
Low-Fat	3 grams of fat (or less) per serving.	Like "fat-Free," this is a good target for you—enjoy!
Reduced-Fat	A minimum of 25 percent less fat, per serving, than the original version.	This really doesn't mean much for higher fat products, so beware this code word—it can be deceptive.
Light	Half the fat, per serving, of the original version.	This may or may not be significant, depending on the fat content of the original, so be sure to check the actual fat grams per serving first.
Lean	Less than 10 grams of fat per serving, including less than 4.5 grams of saturated fat, and less than 95 milligrams of cholesterol.	Not bad, but not great. Use this only if you can't get Extra-Lean.
Extra Lean	Less than 5 grams of fat per serving, and less than 95 milligrams of cholesterol	FYI—when it comes to meats, this is the good stuff. Get it if you can.

Cheat Sheet:
Restaurant Code Words
(part one)

Code Word	What It Means	Advice
Alfredo	Cheese & cream-based sauce	Avoid
Au Gratin	Food covered with cheese or bread crumbs and butter	Avoid
Au Jus	The drippings or juice from the meat. Usually no fat is added (although it may contain some fat from the meat); used as an alternative to gravy	Enjoy!
Baked	Oven-Cooked using dry heat	Enjoy! But instruct your server not to use any butter or dairy, or oil-based marinade on your baked food
Blanched	The food has been dropped into boiling water, then quickly plunged into cold water. It's a fast way of cooking that keeps foods (typically vegetables) crunchy and can remove unwanted peelings as well	Enjoy!
Braised	Slowly cooked in a tightly covered pan	Enjoy! But ask your server to remove any excess fat separated out by the braising process
Broiled	Cooked under an overhead heat source	Enjoy! But instruct your server not to use any butter or dairy or oil-based marinade on your baked food
Buttery	Hey Dude, this doesn't mean it just tastes like butter. It means there really is butter in it!	Avoid
Creamed (also, Creamy, or In Cream Sauce)	Cream and butter are added to your food	Avoid
Crisped	Fried in oil	Avoid

Cheat Sheet:
Restaurant Code Words
(part two)

Code Word	What It Means	Advice
Fried (also, Pan-Fried, Oven-Fried, Lightly-Fried, etc.)	Fried in oil	Avoid
Grilled	Cooked over an open flame (this allows some fat to liquefy and drip off your food).	Enjoy! but instruct your server not to use any butter or dairy or oil-based marinade on your grilled food
Hollandaise Sauce (or any sauce that ends in "aise")	Your food is covered in a sauce made mostly of egg yolks and butter	Avoid
Loaded	High-fat ingredients have been added to your food (such as butter, bacon, sour cream, cheese, and so on).	Avoid
Poached	Your food is boiled, steamed, or simmered in water	Enjoy!
Roasted	Usually means baked, but marinades, oils, or cream-based gravies may have been poured over during the cooking process	Enjoy! But instruct your server not to use any butter or dairy, or oil-based marinade, or added gravies on your roasted food
Sautéed	Cooked in butter or oil	Avoid
Steamed	Cooked over (but not in) boiling water; a particularly flavorful way to prepare rice and other vegetables, along with some meats	Enjoy!
Tender	Usually refers to meat with high fat content	Avoid

As you can see, even if a food is prepared in a desirable manner, the restaurant can thwart your good intentions by adding butter or dairy or oil to your food!

I've been disappointed more than once to find my steamed broccoli had been covered with butter before being brought to my table. I've learned it's very important to talk to your server and ask for further clarification before ordering. Even if you've figured out how to skip sautéed vegetables and choose grilled ones instead, if a spoonful of oil is ladled over the top, you're good plans just went out the window. Eater Beware!

Best Choices for Fast-Food* [94]

	Menu Item	Special Requests	Total Fat (in grams)
Arby's	Ham & Swiss Melt		8
	Jr. Roast Beef Sandwich	no mayonnaise	9
Burger King	BK Fresh Apple Fries		0
	BK Veggie Burger	no mayonnaise	7
	TenderGrill Chicken Sandwich	no mayonnaise	7
	TenderGrill Garden Salad	with Fat-Free Ranch Dressing	7
	Egg only Croissan'wich		12
	Whopper Jr	no mayonnaise	10
	BK Big Fish	no tartar sauce	12
Carl's Jr.	Original Grilled Chicken Salad	no dressing	6
	Charbroiled BBQ Chicken		12
	Kid's Hamburger		10
	Cranberry, Apple, Walnut, Grilled Chicken Salad	no dressing	11
Chick-fil-A	Chargrilled Chicken Sandwich	no dressing	3.5
	IceDream Cone		4
	Chargrilled Chicken and Fruit Salad		6
	Chargrilled Chicken Garden Salad		6
	Southwest Chargrilled Chicken Salad		9
	Chargrilled Chicken Club Sandwich	no mayonnaise	12
	Spicy Chicken Cool Wrap	no dressing	12

*__Note__: Fast-food menus change frequently. Be sure to check the appropriate menu online to verify the information in this chart.

Best Choices for Fast-Food*
(continued)

	Menu Item	Special Requests	Total Fat (in grams)
Chipotle	Chicken Burrito Bowl	with black or pinto beans, cilantro-lime rice, lettuce, and tomato or green tomatillo salsa—no cheese or sour cream	10.5
	Steak Burrito Bowl	with black or pinto beans, cilantro-lime rice, lettuce, and tomato or green tomatillo salsa—no cheese or sour cream	10.5
Domino's Pizza	1 Slice from a 12" Feast Deep Dish pizza	"America's Favorite Feast" version	5 (per slice)
	1 Slice from a 12" hand-tossed pizza	with one of the following toppings: Cheese only; Ham only; Ham and Pineapple; Green Peppers, Onion, and Mushrooms	6 (per slice)
	1 Slice from a 12" hand-tossed pizza	with Pepperoni only	8 (per slice)
	1 Slice from a 12" hand-tossed pizza	with one of the following toppings: Beef only; Sausage only	9 (per slice)
Einstein Bros. Bagels	Café Latte, non-fat		1
	Blueberry Bagel, or Everything Bagel, or Honey Whole Wheat Bagel	no cream cheese; no butter	2 (each bagel)
	Chocolate Chip Bagel, or Cinnamon Sugar Chicago Style Bagel, or Garlic Dip'd Bagel, or Onion Dip'd Bagel	no cream cheese; no butter	2.5 (each bagel)
	Sesame Dip'd Bagel, or Poppy Dip'd Bagel	no cream cheese; no butter	3 (each bagel)

*__Note__: *Fast-food menus change frequently. Be sure to check the appropriate menu online to verify the information in this chart.*

Dude, You Don't Have to be Fat

Best Choices for Fast-Food*
(continued)

	Menu Item	Special Requests	Total Fat (in grams)
Einstein Bros. Bagels	Asiago Cheese Bagel, or Fruit and Nut Power Bagel, or Egg Bagel	no cream cheese; no butter	5 (per bagel)
	Reduced Fat Whipped Cream Cheese (various flavors)		5
	Six-Cheese Gourmet Bagel		6
	Dutch Apple Gourmet Bagel		7
	Green Chile or Spinach Florentine Gourmet Bagel		8 (each bagel)
Firehouse Subs	Turkey Sub	no mayonnaise; no cheese	4
	Engineer Sub	no mayonnaise; no cheese	5
	Veggie Sub	no mayonnaise; no cheese	5
	Engine Company Sub	no mayonnaise; no cheese	6
	Roast Beef Sub	no mayonnaise; no cheese	6
	Ham Sub	no mayonnaise; no cheese	7
	Hero Sub	no mayonnaise; no cheese	7
	Hook and Ladder Sub	no mayonnaise; no cheese	7
In-N-Out Burger	Hamburger	with onion, ketchup, and mustard—but no spread	10
Jack in the Box	Fruit Smoothie	Mango, or Strawberry, or Strawberry-Banana, or Tropical	0
	Chicken Teriyaki Bowl		6
	Grilled Chicken Strips (4)		6

***Note**: Fast-food menus change frequently. Be sure to check the appropriate menu online to verify the information in this chart.*

Mike Nappa

Best Choices for Fast-Food*
(continued)

	Menu Item	Special Requests	Total Fat (in grams)
Jack in the Box	Chocolate Overload Cake		7
	Egg Roll (1)		7
	Grilled Chicken Salad		8
	Breakfast Jack		11
	Chicken Fajita Pita	no salsa	11
	Steak Teriyaki Bowl		11
KFC	Grilled Chicken Caesar Salad	no dressing, no croutons	7
	Original Chicken Filet (3.5 ounces)		7
	Grilled Chicken BLT Salad	no dressing, no croutons	8
	Grilled Chicken Breast		8
McDonald's	Apple Dippers with Low-Fat Caramel Dip		0.5
	McCafe Smoothies (all fruit flavors)		1
	Fruit 'n Yogurt Parfait		2
	Vanilla Reduced Fat Ice Cream Cone		3.5
	Premium Caesar Salad	no Chicken	4
	Fruit and Maple Oatmeal		4
	Premium Southwest Salad	no Chicken	4.5
	Premium Caesar Salad	with Grilled Chicken	6
	Egg White Delight McMuffin		8
	Hamburger		9
	Honey Mustard Snack Wrap (Grilled)		9
	Chipotle BBQ Snack Wrap (Grilled)		9

***Note**: Fast-food menus change frequently. Be sure to check the appropriate menu online to verify the information in this chart.

Dude, You Don't Have to be Fat

Best Choices for Fast-Food*
(continued)

	Menu Item	Special Requests	Total Fat (in grams)
McDonald's	Hotcakes, with syrup	no butter	9
	Premium Grilled Chicken Classic Sandwich		9
	Premium Southwest Salad with Grilled Chicken		9
	Premium Grilled Chicken Ranch BLT Sandwich		10
	Ranch Snack Wrap (Grilled)		10
	Egg McMuffin		12
Panda Express	Mixed Veggies (side dish)		0.5
	Fortune Cookies		2
	Hot and Sour Soup		3.5
	Veggie Spring Roll (1)		3.5
	Broccoli Beef, with steamed rice		6
	Kobari Beef, with steamed rice		7
	String Bean Chicken Breast, with steamed rice		7
	Mongolian Beef, with steamed rice		11
	Potato Chicken, with steamed rice		11
Papa Murphy's	1 Slice Thin Crust deLITE Cheese Pizza		7 (per slice)
	1 Slice Thin Crust deLITE Hawaiian Pizza		7 (per slice)
	1 Slice Thin Crust deLITE Pepperoni Pizza		9 (per slice)

***Note**: Fast-food menus change frequently. Be sure to check the appropriate menu online to verify the information in this chart.*

Best Choices for Fast-Food*
(continued)

	Menu Item	Special Requests	Total Fat (in grams)
Papa Murphy's	1 Slice Thin Crust deLITE Veggie Pizza		9 (per slice)
Pizza Hut	1 Slice from a 12" Fit 'n Delicious Green Pepper, Onion, and Tomato Pizza		4 (per slice)
	1 Slice from a 12" Fit 'n Delicious Tomato, Mushroom, and Jalapeno Pizza		4.5 (per slice)
	1 Slice from a 12" Fit 'n Delicious Chicken, Mushroom, and Jalapeno Pizza		4.5 (per slice)
	1 Slice from a 12" Fit 'n Delicious Chicken, Onion, and Green Pepper		4.5 (per slice)
	1 Slice from a 12" Fit 'n Delicious Ham, Onion, and Mushroom Pizza		4.5 (per slice)
	1 Slice from a 12" Fit 'n Delicious Ham, Pineapple, and Tomato Pizza		4.5 (per slice)
	1 Slice from a 12" Thin 'n Crispy, Cheese Only Pizza		6 (per slice)
	1 Slice from a 12" Thin 'n Crispy, Ham and Pineapple Pizza		6 (per slice)
	1 Slice from a 12" Thin 'n Crispy, Veggie Lover's Pizza		6 (per slice)
	1 Slice from a 12" Hand-Tossed Style, Ham and Pineapple Pizza		7 (per slice)

***Note**: Fast-food menus change frequently. Be sure to check the appropriate menu online to verify the information in this chart.*

Best Choices for Fast-Food*
(continued)

	Menu Item	Special Requests	Total Fat (in grams)
Pizza Hut	1 Slice from a 12" Hand-Tossed Style, Veggie Lover's Pizza		7 (per slice)
	1 Slice from a 12" Pizza Mia, Cheese and Pepperoni Pizza		7.5 (per slice)
	1 Slice from a 12" Hand-Tossed Style, Cheese Only Pizza		8 (per slice)
	1 Slice from a 12" Hand-Tossed Style, Pepperoni and Mushroom Pizza		8 (per slice)
	1 Slice from a 12" Pan Style, Veggie Lover's Pizza		9 (per slice)
	1 Slice from a 12" Pan Style, Ham and Pineapple Pizza		9 (per slice)
Starbucks		Always ask for non-fat milk or creamer in any coffee drink at Starbucks!	
	Deluxe Fruit Blend Salad		0
	Plain Bagel		1
	Starbucks Perfect Oatmeal		2.5
	Strawberry & Blueberry Yogurt Parfait		3.5
	Dark Cherry Yogurt Parfait		4
	Marshmallow Dream Bar		4
	Multigrain Bagel		4
	Asiago Bagel		4.5
	Chonga Bagel		5
	Petite Vanilla Bean Scone		5

***Note**: Fast-food menus change frequently. Be sure to check the appropriate menu online to verify the information in this chart.*

Best Choices for Fast-Food*
(continued)

	Menu Item	Special Requests	Total Fat (in grams)
Starbucks	Birthday Cake Mini Doughnut		6
	Double Fudge Mini Doughnut		7
	Reduced-Fat Banana Chocolate Chip Coffee Cake		7
	Reduced-Fat Turkey Bacon with Egg Whites on English Muffin		7
	8-Grain Roll		8
	Chicken & Hummus Bistro Box		8
	Hawaiian Bagel		8
	Apple Bran Muffin		9
	Chicken on Flatbread with Hummus Artisan Snack Plate		9
	Reduced-Fat Cinnamon Swirl Coffee Cake		9
	Egg White, Spinach & Feta Wrap		10
	Reduced-Fat Very Berry Coffee Cake		10
	Snack-Fulls		10
Subway	Apple Slices		0
	Tomato Garden Vegetable Soup with Rotini		0.5
	Fire Roasted Tomato Orzo Soup		1
	Minestrone Soup		1
	Chicken Tortilla Soup		1.5
	Rosemary Chicken and Dumpling Soup		1.5

***Note**: *Fast-food menus change frequently. Be sure to check the appropriate menu online to verify the information in this chart.*

Best Choices for Fast-Food*
(continued)

	Menu Item	Special Requests	Total Fat (in grams)
Subway	Roasted Chicken Noodle Soup		2
	Vegetable Beef Soup		2
	Six-Inch Veggie Delite Sub Sandwich	no cheese, no oil, no mayonnaise	2.5
	Spanish Style Chicken Soup with Rice		2.5
	Chipotle Chicken Corn Chowder		3
	Six-Inch Turkey Breast Sub Sandwich	no cheese, no oil, no mayonnaise	3.5
	Six-Inch Turkey Breast & Black Forest Ham Sub Sandwich	no cheese, no oil, no mayonnaise	4
	Six-Inch Black Forest Ham Sub Sandwich	no cheese, no oil, no mayonnaise	4.5
	Six-Inch Oven-Roasted Chicken Breast Sub Sandwich	no cheese, no oil, no mayonnaise	4.5
	Six-Inch Roast Beef Sub Sandwich	no cheese, no oil, no mayonnaise	4.5
	Six-Inch Sweet Onion Chicken Teriyaki Sub Sandwich	no cheese, no oil, no mayonnaise	4.5
	Chicken and Dumpling Soup		5
	New England Style Clam Chowder		5
	Six-Inch Subway Club Sub Sandwich	no cheese, no oil, no mayonnaise	5
	Six-Inch Veggie Delite Sub Sandwich	no cheese, no oil, no mayonnaise	5
	Flatbread Turkey Breast Sandwich	no cheese, no oil, no mayonnaise	6
	Flatbread Black Forest Ham Sandwich	no cheese, no oil, no mayonnaise	7
	Flatbread Sweet Onion Chicken Teriyaki Sandwich	no cheese, no oil, no mayonnaise	7

*__Note__: Fast-food menus change frequently. Be sure to check the appropriate menu online to verify the information in this chart.

Best Choices for Fast-Food*
(continued)

	Menu Item	Special Requests	Total Fat (in grams)
Subway	Flatbread Turkey Breast & Black Forest Ham Sandwich	no cheese, no oil, no mayonnaise	7
	Flatbread Oven-Roasted Chicken Breast Sandwich	no cheese, no oil, no mayonnaise	8
	Flatbread Roast Beef Sandwich	no cheese, no oil, no mayonnaise	8
	Flatbread Subway Club Sandwich	no cheese, no oil, no mayonnaise	8
Taco Bell	Chicken Soft Taco	Fresco Style	3.5
	Grilled Steak Soft Taco	Fresco Style	4
	Chicken Soft Taco		6
	Cinnamon Twists		7
	Crunchy Taco	Fresco Style	7
	Beef Soft Taco	Fresco Style	7
	Bean Burrito	Fresco Style	8
	Burrito Supreme – Chicken	Fresco Style	8
	Burrito Supreme – Steak	Fresco Style	8
	Cheese Roll-Up		9
	Beef Soft Taco		9
	Tostada		10
Wendy's	Plain Baked Potato	with Fat-Free Ranch Dressing	0
	Sour Cream and Chives Baked Potato		3.5
	Chocolate Frosty, Small		6
	Chili with Saltine Crackers Small / Large		6.5 / 9.5
	Ultimate Chicken Grill Sandwich	no mayonnaise	7

__Note__: Fast-food menus change frequently. Be sure to check the appropriate menu online to verify the information in this chart.

Best Choices for Fast-Food*
(continued)

	Menu Item	Special Requests	Total Fat (in grams)
Wendy's	Vanilla Frosty, Small	Regular or with Coca-Cola	7
	Hamburger	no mayonnaise	8
	Caramel Apple Parfait		9
	Grilled Chicken Go Wrap		10
	Apple Pecan Chicken Salad		11

***Note**: Fast-food menus change frequently. Be sure to check the appropriate menu online to verify the information in this chart.

Best Choices at Fine-Dining Restaurants*

	Menu Item	Special Requests	Total Fat (in grams)
Applebees	Chicken Noodle Soup		3
	Weight Watchers® Paradise Chicken Salad		4
	Grilled Shrimp and Island Rice		4.5
	Weight Watchers® Cajun Lime Tilapia		5
	Weight Watchers® Spicy Pineapple Glazed Shrimp & Spinach		5
	Chicken Tortilla Soup		7
	Teriyaki Shrimp Pasta		8
	Teriyaki Chicken Pasta		8
	Black Bean Soup		9
	Grilled Chicken Caesar Salad	no dressing	10
	7 oz. House Sirloin Steak	Order fresh fruit or seasonal vegetables, no butter, for a zero-fat side dish	12
	Weight Watchers® Chipotle Lime Chicken		12
	Weight Watchers® Steak & Potato Salad		12
	Asiago Peppercorn Steak	try ordering without cheese for lower fat count	12
Chili's	Chicken & Green Chile Soup (Bowl)		7

*Note: Restaurant menus change regularly. Be sure to check the appropriate menu online to verify the information in this chart.

Best Choices at Fine-Dining Restaurants* [95]
(continued)

	Menu Item	Special Requests	Total Fat (in grams)
Chili's	Margarita Grilled Chicken	Order fresh fruit or seasonal vegetables, no butter, for a zero-fat side dish	7
	Spicy Garlic & Lime Grilled Shrimp	Order fresh fruit or seasonal vegetables, no butter, for a zero-fat side dish	8
	GG Classic Sirloin, with Steamed Broccoli		9
	Chicken Fajitas	no tortillas, no condiments	10
Denny's	Egg-White Veggie Omelet	no butter, no cheese	1
	Vegetable Beef Soup		1
	Chicken Noodle Soup		4
	Buttermilk Pancakes (3), with maple syrup	no butter	6
	Cranberry Chicken Pecan Salad	no dressing	8
	Grilled Chicken Deluxe Salad	no dressing	10
	Grilled Shrimp Skewers		10
	Fit Fare Grilled Tilapia		11
Don Pablo's	Tortilla Salad	no dressing, no shell	5
	Chicken Tamale		6
	Mama's Skinny Enchilada		7
	White Chicken Chili (Bowl)		11
	Tortilla Soup (Bowl)		12
	Grilled Tilapia		12

***Note**: Restaurant menus change regularly. Be sure to check the appropriate menu online to verify the information in this chart.

Best Choices at Fine-Dining Restaurants*
(continued)

	Menu Item	Special Requests	Total Fat (in grams)
Don Pablo's	Chicken Relleno		13
	Chicken Soft Taco		13
	Lunch Sized Chicken Fajitas		13
Golden Corral	Flame Broiled Mixed Vegetables		0
	Chicken Breast, Cooked (1)		2.5
	Hickory Bourbon Chicken Breast (1)		3.5
	Boneless Spiral Cut Ham (3oz)		4
	Fajita Chicken (3 oz)		4
	Awesome Pot Roast (3 oz)		4.5
	Baked New Orleans Style Fish		5
	Beef Tips, Marinated (3 oz)		5
	Brazilian Carved Churrasco Steak (3 oz)		6
	Breaded Bay Scallops (10)		6
	Fajita Steak (3 oz)		6
	Hickory Bourbon Chicken Tenders (3)		6
	Machaca Chicken (3 oz)		6
	Peppercorn London Broil (3 oz, about 2 slices)		6
	Popcorn Shrimp (15)		6
	Red Beans and Rice (1/2 cup)		6

*Note: Restaurant menus change regularly. Be sure to check the appropriate menu online to verify the information in this chart.

Dude, You Don't Have to be Fat

Best Choices at Fine-Dining Restaurants*
(continued)

	Menu Item	Special Requests	Total Fat (in grams)
Golden Corral	Salmon, Whole Carved (3 oz)		6
	Tortellini and Shrimp in Lobster Sauce (1/2 cup)		6
	Cheese Pizza (1 slice)		7
	Chipotle Chicken Breast (1)		7
	Clam Strips (10)		7
	Spicy Glazed Habanero Shrimp (18)		7
	Teriyaki Beef (1 cup)		7
	Whole Carved Turkey (White Meat w/ skin) (3 oz)		7
	BBQ Pork (3 oz)		8
	Beef Quesadilla (1)		8
	Jalapeno Glazed Tilapia (1)		8
	Machaca Beef (3 oz)		8
	Oriental Pepper Beef (1 cup)		8
	Asian Beef (1 cup)		9
	Bourbon Street Chicken (3oz)		9
	Buffalo Shrimp (6)		9
	Golden Delicious Shrimp (6)		9
	Macaroni and Cheese (1/2 cup)		9
	Sirloin (4.5 oz)		9

***Note**: Restaurant menus change regularly. Be sure to check the appropriate menu online to verify the information in this chart.

Best Choices at Fine-Dining Restaurants*
(continued)

	Menu Item	Special Requests	Total Fat (in grams)
Golden Corral	Baked Fish with Shrimp and Lemon Herb Sauce		10
	Mongolian Beef (1 cup)		10
	North Carolina BBQ Pork (3 oz)		10
	Panko Shrimp (6)		10
	Salmon Lemonata (3 oz)		10
	Spaghetti Bake (1/2 cup)		10
	Spicy Sweet Pagoda Chicken (1 cup)		10
	Sweet and Sour Chicken (1 cup)		10
	Bacon Wrapped Sirloin (1)	Take the bacon off before you eat this!	11
	Beef Enchilada (1)		11
	Breaded Catfish (2 pieces)		11
	Sweet and Sour Pork (1 cup)		11
	Sweet and Sour Shrimp (1 cup)		11
	Baked Florentine Fish		12
	Chicken Parmesan (1)		12
	Coconut Shrimp (5)		12
International House of Pancakes (IHOP)	Minestrone Soup		2
	SIMPLE & FIT Fresh Fruit & Yogurt Bowl		3

*Note: Restaurant menus change regularly. Be sure to check the appropriate menu online to verify the information in this chart.

Best Choices at Fine-Dining Restaurants*
(continued)

	Menu Item	Special Requests	Total Fat (in grams)
IHOP	Create Your Own Omelette: Plain with Egg Substitute		4
	Create Your Own Omelette: Egg Substitute with Green Peppers, Onions, Tomatoes, Spinach, and/or Mushrooms		4
	House Salad with Reduced-Fat Italian Dressing		4
	SIMPLE & FIT Oatmeal		4.5
	Chicken Noodle Soup		5
	Create Your Own Omelette: Egg Substitute with Diced Ham		5
	Create Your Own Omelette, Egg Substitute with Diced Ham		8
	SIMPLE & FIT Two-Egg Breakfast		8
	SIMPLE & FIT Simply Chicken Sandwich w/ Fresh Fruit		9
Lone Star Steakhouse	Mesquite Grilled Shrimp Dinner		2
	Mesquite Grilled Chicken		2.5
	Grilled Chicken Caesar Salad	no dressing	10
	Mesquite Grilled Sweet Bourbon Salmon		11
Olive Garden	Minestrone Soup		1.5

Note: *Restaurant menus change regularly. Be sure to check the appropriate menu online to verify the information in this chart.*

Best Choices at Fine-Dining Restaurants*
(continued)

	Menu Item	Special Requests	Total Fat (in grams)
Olive Garden	Breadstick with garlic-butter spread (1)	If you ask, Olive Garden will happily bake fresh breadsticks with no butter spread on them ... but you have to ask	2
	Pasta e Fagioli Soup		2
	Famous House Salad (one serving)	with low-fat dressing	4
	Venetian Apricot Chicken (lunch serving)		4
	Zuppa Toscana Soup		4
	Venetian Apricot Chicken (dinner serving)		7
	Spaghetti with Meat Sauce Mini Pasta Bowl (lunch serving)		9
	Shrimp Primavera (lunch serving)		9
	Spaghetti with Traditional Marina Sauce and Grilled Chicken Topping (dinner serving)		10.5
	Capellini Pomodoro (lunch serving)		11
	Shrimp Primavera (dinner serving)		12
	Spaghetti with Traditional Marina Sauce and Grilled Chicken Topping (dinner serving)		14
On the Border Mexican Grill	Achiote Chicken Taco		4

***Note**: Restaurant menus change regularly. Be sure to check the appropriate menu online to verify the information in this chart.*

Dude, You Don't Have to be Fat

Best Choices at Fine-Dining Restaurants*
(continued)

	Menu Item	Special Requests	Total Fat (in grams)
On the Border Mexican Grill	Citrus Chipotle Chicken Salad w/ Mango Citrus Vinaigrette		4
	Chicken Tostada		5
	Black Beans and Mexican Rice		8
	Chicken Salsa Fresca		9
	Ground Beef Tostada		9
	Chicken Enchilada with Sour Cream Sauce		11
	Chicken Soft Taco		11
Outback Steakhouse	Lobster Tails with Fresh Seasonal Veggies and Sweet Potato	no butter on anything	6.5
	Grilled Chicken on the Barbie, with Fresh Seasonal Veggies no butter on anything	no butter on anything	8.5
	Teriyaki Marinated Sirloin and Fresh Seasonal Veggies	no butter on anything	12
P.F. Chang's China Bistro	Buddha's Feast – Steamed, on: White Rice or Brown Rice		1 or 2
	Spring Roll (1)		4
	P.F. Chang's Vegetable Fried Rice		5
	Asian Grilled Norwegian Salmon on: White Rice or Brown Rice		5 or 6
	Chang's Chicken Lettuce Wraps		7

*Note: Restaurant menus change regularly. Be sure to check the appropriate menu online to verify the information in this chart.

Best Choices at Fine-Dining Restaurants*
(continued)

	Menu Item	Special Requests	Total Fat (in grams)
P.F. Chang's China Bistro	Chang's Vegetarian Lettuce Wraps		7
	Sichuan Shrimp		7
	Ginger Chicken with Broccoli		11
	Moo Goo Gai Pan on White Rice		11
	Salt & Pepper Prawns		11
	Shrimp with Lobster Sauce on: White Rice or Brown Rice		11 or 12
	Beef A La Sichuan		12
	Beef with Broccoli on White Rice		12
	Chengdu Spiced Lamb		12
	Pepper Steak on White Rice		12
Red Lobster	Live Maine Lobster, Steamed		0
	Chilled Jumbo Shrimp Cocktail		0.5
	Manhattan Clam Chowder		1
	Corvina, or Flounder, or Grouper, or Haddock, or Mahi Mahi, or Monchong, or Gulf Snapper, Wood-Grilled, Broiled or Blackened, with Broccoli	half portion	1.5
	Rockzilla		1.5

Note: Restaurant menus change regularly. Be sure to check the appropriate menu online to verify the information in this chart.

Dude, You Don't Have to be Fat

Best Choices at Fine-Dining Restaurants*
(continued)

	Menu Item	Special Requests	Total Fat (in grams)
Red Lobster	Cod, or Halibut, or Perch, or Sole, or Walleye, Wood-Grilled, Broiled or Blackened, with Broccoli	half portion	2
	Lake Whitefish, or Red Rockfish, or Ono/Wahoo, Wood-Grilled, Broiled or Blackened, with Broccoli	half portion	2.5
	Tilapia, Wood-Grilled or Broiled, with Broccoli	half portion	3
	North Pacific King Crab Legs		3.5
	Barramundi, Wood-Grilled, Broiled or Blackened, with Broccoli	half portion	5
	Seafood-Stuffed Flounder		5
	Seabass, Wood-Grilled, Broiled or Blackened, with Broccoli	half portion	6
	Pompano, Wood-Grilled, Broiled or Blackened, with Broccoli	half portion	8
	Seafood Gumbo		8
	Garlic-Grilled Jumbo Shrimp		9
	Maple-Glazed Chicken		9
	Salmon, Wood-Grilled or Broiled, with Broccoli	half portion	9

__Note__: Restaurant menus change regularly. Be sure to check the appropriate menu online to verify the information in this chart.

Best Choices at Fine-Dining Restaurants*
(continued)

	Menu Item	Special Requests	Total Fat (in grams)
Red Lobster	Broiled Seafood Platter		10
	Rainbow Trout, Wood-Grilled or Broiled, with Broccoli	half portion	10
Red Robin	Vegan Boca Burger	no country Dijon spread	5
	Blackened Chicken Sandwich	no mayonnaise, no cheese	7
	Ensenada Chicken Platter, 1 Piece	no cheese, no dressing	7
	Garden Burger	no country Dijon spread	7
	Grilled Salmon Sandwich	no country Dijon spread	7
	Teriyaki Chicken Sandwich	no mayonnaise, no cheese	7
	Simply Grilled Chicken Sandwich		8
	Ensenada Chicken Platter, 2 Piece	no cheese and no dressing	9
Romano's Macaroni Grill	Jumbo Shrimp Spiedini		7
	Grilled Chicken Spiedini		9
	1/2 Grilled Chicken Sandwich		10
	1/2 Imported Prosciutto Sandwich		11
	Aged Beef Tenderloin Spiedini		12
	Amalfi Chicken Soup		12
Ruby Tuesday	Plain Grilled Chicken		4
	Barbecue Grilled Chicken, Fit & Trim		4

***Note**: Restaurant menus change regularly. Be sure to check the appropriate menu online to verify the information in this chart.*

Dude, You Don't Have to be Fat

Best Choices at Fine-Dining Restaurants*
(continued)

	Menu Item	Special Requests	Total Fat (in grams)
Ruby Tuesday	Plain Grilled Petite Sirloin		6
	Creole Catch		8
	White Bean Chicken Chili		8
	Mango Chicken and Jumbo Garlic Shrimp		9
	Plain Grilled Salmon		11
	Plain Grilled Top Sirloin		12

*__Note__: Restaurant menus change regularly. Be sure to check the appropriate menu online to verify the information in this chart.

Recommended Resources

* = Highly Recommended

Books

American Heart Association. *Low-Fat, Low-Cholesterol Cookbook, Fourth Edition*
Bob Greene, *The Best Life Diet*
Chef Devin Alexander et.al., *The Biggest Loser Family Cookbook*
*Cooking Light What to Eat**
David Zinczenko, *The Abs Diet Ultimate Nutrition Handbook*
Dean Ornish, M.D. *Eat More, Weigh Less**
Jackie Warner, *This is Why You're Fat*
Joseph C. Piscatella, *Fat-Proof Your Child*
Julia Greer, MD, MPH, *The Anti-Cancer Cookbook*
Lisa Dorfman with Sandra J. Gordon, *The Reunion Diet*
Louis J. Aronne, M.D., *The Skinny on Losing Weight without Being Hungry**
Lynn Fischer, *Fabulous Fat-Free Cooking*
Molly Morgan, RD, CDN, *The Skinny Rules*
Phyllis Pellman Good, *Fix-It and Forget-It Lightly*
Robert K. Cooper, Ph.D., with Leslie L. Cooper, *Low-Fat Living*
Steven Sinatra, M.D. and James Punkre, *The Fast Food Diet*
Taste of Home, *Guilt-Free Cooking*
*The Calorie King Calorie, Fat, and Carbohydrate Counter**
The Special K Challenge and Beyond
Weight Watchers New Complete Cookbook
William Sears, M.D. and Martha Sears, R.N., *The Family Nutrition Book*

Magazines

Cooking Light
Fitness RX for Men
Men's Fitness
Men's Health
On Fitness
Weight Watchers
Whole Living

Websites

10poundsdown.com
americanheart.org
calorieking.com
choosemyplate.gov
coloradohealthnutrition.com
cookinglight.com
dietfacts.com
fatsecret.com
goodfoodnearyou.com

healthcentral.com
healthy-eating.com
healthychoice.com
internethealthlibrary.com
jessicasmith.tv
leancuisine.com
livestrong.com
livingthin.com
naturalnews.com
skinnycow.com
sparkpeople.com
sunriseriverpress.com
surgeongeneral.gov
webmd.com
yourlife.usatoday.com/health/index

Other

10 Minute Solution: Ultimate Bootcamp DVD with Jessica Smith
Look Better Naked Workout DVD with Jessica Smith
Richard H. Carmona, M.D., M.P.H., F.A.C.S. "The Obesity Crisis in America." Office of the Surgeon General
U.S. Department of Agriculture and U.S. Department of Health and Human Services. *Dietary Guidelines for Americans, 2010. 7th Edition*

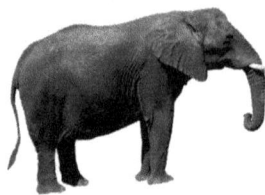

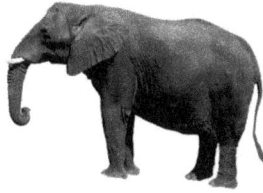

Part 5

Mini-Cookbook
for Men

Special thanks to Livestrong.org for calculating the Nutrition Facts for the recipes in this section! [96]

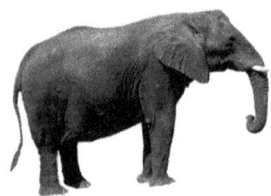

Breakfast
10 easy recipes for delicious day-starters

Banana Chocolate Milkshake

This one's for guys who prefer a lighter breakfast—but a full stomach—to start the day off right.

1 to 2 frozen bananas (about 5 to 10 frozen chunks)
1 tablespoon fat-free chocolate syrup
1 cup skim milk

Peel your banana(s) and break them into bite-size chunks. Combine all ingredients in a blender, and purify until smooth. Add additional banana chunks as desired. (For a thicker milkshake, use up to two bananas; for a normal milkshake, use one.)

Note:
If you like, you can also add fat-free strawberry syrup to the mix to create a Strawberry-Banana Chocolate Milkshake.

Serves: 1
Total Fat Content Per Serving: 0

Nutrition Facts

1 servings per container

Serving size	1 shake

Amount Per Serving

Calories	360

	% Daily Value*
Total Fat 0g	0%
Saturated Fat 0g	0%
Trans Fat 0g	
Cholesterol < 5mg	2%
Sodium 140mg	6%
Total Carbohydrate 82g	30%
Dietary Fiber 8g	30%
Total Sugars 66g	
Includes 0g Added Sugars	0%
Protein 11g	22%

Not a significant source of vitamin D, calcium, iron, and potassium

* The % Daily Value (DV) tells you how much a nutrient in a serving of food contributes to a daily diet. 2,000 calories a day is used for general nutrition advice.

Tip:
If you break your banana into chunks before you freeze, it's a lot easier to work with. Break up a bunch of bananas and put them into a re-sealable plastic bag, toss them in the freezer, and you'll always have frozen chunks available. Win!

Big'n's Breakfast Burrito

Great for a Saturday morning, or when you want to plan ahead for the week.

1/2 cup Egg Beaters (equivalent to two large eggs)
1 slice Jennie-O Lean Turkey Bacon
2 tablespoons Kraft Natural Shredded Fat Free Cheddar Cheese
1 low-fat or no-fat flour tortilla (such as Mission brand or Olé Mexican Foods brand low-fat or no-fat tortillas)
Black pepper (optional) and/or Mrs. Dash Table Blend (optional)

Scramble Egg Beaters in a skillet, seasoning to taste with black pepper and/or Mrs. Dash Table Blend. Cook turkey bacon according to instructions on package.

Spread scrambled Egg Beaters in tortilla and crumble bacon onto tortilla as well. Sprinkle with cheese, and then fold tortilla burrito-style. Enjoy fresh and warm, or freeze for future use.

Note:
For a less-stuffed version of this breakfast burrito, cut all filling amounts in half.

Serves: 1
Total Fat Content Per Serving: 4 grams

Nutrition Facts

1 servings per container

Serving size	**1 burrito**

Amount Per Serving

Calories	**260**

	% Daily Value*
Total Fat 4g	**5%**
Saturated Fat 0.5g	**3%**
Trans Fat 0g	
Cholesterol 10mg	**3%**
Sodium 690mg	**30%**
Total Carbohydrate 30g	**11%**
Dietary Fiber 3g	**11%**
Total Sugars 4g	
Includes 0g Added Sugars	**0%**
Protein 27g	**54%**

Not a significant source of vitamin D, calcium, iron, and potassium

*The % Daily Value (DV) tells you how much a nutrient in a serving of food contributes to a daily diet. 2,000 calories a day is used for general nutrition advice.

Tip:
Make up several of these and freeze them individually. Heat one in a microwave for about 1-2 minutes you'll have a tasty, quick-prep breakfast you can eat on your way to work.

Cinnamon Crunch Coffee Cake

Super fast and great for a Sunday morning.

1 cup sugar
2 cups flour
2 teaspoons baking powder
1 tablespoon vegetable oil
1 ½ cups skim milk

For topping
2 tablespoons sugar
2 teaspoons cinnamon

Mix dry ingredients together in a bowl. Mix oil in milk in separate bowl, and then stir together with the dry ingredients. Pour everything into a 9x9 baking pan that you've lightly coated with cooking spray.

Mix the remaining sugar and cinnamon together and sprinkle over top of the uncooked batter. Bake at 350 degrees for 35-40 minutes, or until a knife inserted into the center of the cake comes out clean.

Eat while warm. Cover leftover cake or it will dry out quickly.

Serves: 9
Total Fat Content Per Serving: 1.5 grams

Nutrition Facts

9 servings per container

Serving size	**1 square**

Amount Per Serving

Calories	310

	% Daily Value*
Total Fat 1.5g	2%
Saturated Fat 0.23g	1%
Trans Fat 0g	
Cholesterol 0mg	0%
Sodium 115mg	5%
Total Carbohydrate 67g	24%
Dietary Fiber 0g	1%
Total Sugars 24g	
Includes 0g Added Sugars	0%
Protein 1g	3%

Not a significant source of vitamin D, calcium, iron, and potassium

* The % Daily Value (DV) tells you how much a nutrient in a serving of food contributes to a daily diet. 2,000 calories a day is used for general nutrition advice.

Egg McGuffey

An oldie, but a goodie—and better-tasting than the fatty fast-food version.

1 English muffin
1/4 cup Egg Beaters (equivalent to one large egg)
1 sandwich-sized slice of fat-free American cheese
1 slice (about 2 oz.) Jennie-O Extra-Lean Turkey Ham
black pepper

Toast the English muffin, and then lay it open-faced on a plate. While muffin is still warm, lay cheese on bottom slice to melt. Lightly coat a skillet with fat-free cooking spray and fry Egg Beaters into an omelet, seasoning to taste with black pepper. Place warm omelet on cheese, add turkey ham, and top with second muffin slice to make sandwich.

Eat warm and fresh!

Serves: 1
Total Fat Content Per Serving: 4 grams

Nutrition Facts

1 servings per container

Serving size   1 McGuffy Sandwich

Amount Per Serving

Calories **240**

	% Daily Value*
Total Fat 4g	**5%**
Saturated Fat 1g	**5%**
Trans Fat 0g	
Cholesterol 30mg	**10%**
Sodium 1150mg	**50%**
Total Carbohydrate 30g	**11%**
Dietary Fiber 1g	**4%**
Total Sugars 4g	
Includes 0g Added Sugars	**0%**
Protein 23g	**46%**

Not a significant source of vitamin D, calcium, iron, and potassium

* The % Daily Value (DV) tells you how much a nutrient in a serving of food contributes to a daily diet. 2,000 calories a day is used for general nutrition advice.

French Toast Sammich

I like to eat this one (without syrup) when I'm on the go—perfect to take in the car when you're late for work or trying to make it to the airport for an early-morning flight

Two slices sourdough bread
1/4 cup Egg Beaters (equivalent to one large egg)
1/4 cup skim milk
1 teaspoon vanilla extract
1 slice Jennie-O Lean Turkey Bacon
fruit slices (optional—such as banana slices, berries, or peaches)
maple syrup (optional)

Cook turkey bacon according to instructions on package.

Next beat Egg Beaters, milk, and vanilla in a bowl until they're thoroughly mixed. Lightly cover a skillet with fat-free cooking spray and place on medium heat. Dip bread slices, one at a time, in the egg mixture, making sure both sides of the bread are soaked. Let excess liquid drip off, and then fry the bread in the skillet until both sides are lightly browned.

Add either bacon slice or fruit filling to make a sandwich. Eat plain or on a plate with maple syrup topping.

Serves: 1
Total Fat Content Per Serving: 2.5 grams

Nutrition Facts

1 servings per container

Serving size   **1 Sammich**

Amount Per Serving

Calories   **530**

	% Daily Value*
Total Fat 2.5g	3%
Saturated Fat 0.5g	3%
Trans Fat 0g	
Cholesterol 10mg	4%
Sodium 770mg	33%
Total Carbohydrate 106g	38%
Dietary Fiber 2g	7%
Total Sugars 54g	
Includes 0g Added Sugars	0%
Protein 18g	36%

Not a significant source of vitamin D, calcium, iron, and potassium

*The % Daily Value (DV) tells you how much a nutrient in a serving of food contributes to a daily diet. 2,000 calories a day is used for general nutrition advice.

Meat-Lover's Omelet

This is a hearty breakfast for a man who likes a little meat on his plate each morning. Delicious!

1/8 lb Extra Lean Ground Beef (96% fat free)
5 slices Hormel Turkey Pepperoni
1 slice Jennie-O Lean Turkey Bacon
1/4 cup Kraft Natural Shredded Fat Free Cheddar Cheese
1/2 cup Egg Beaters (equivalent to two large eggs)
2 slices sourdough bread (optional)
1 chopped tomato (optional)

Brown ground beef in a skillet, seasoning as desired. While beef is browning, chop pepperoni into bits. Also cook bacon in microwave. When beef is cooked, turn down the heat on the stove burner to medium, and pour Egg Beaters into skillet. Stir in cheese and chopped pepperoni, and let omelet cook on the bottom. When edges appear firm, fold omelet in half and cook 30 seconds to a minute more. Then flip omelet over and cook to desired consistency.

Transfer cooked omelet to plate, and crumble bacon into bits over the top. (Optional) spread chopped tomato chunks over the top too.

Serve with (optional) dry sourdough toast and enjoy!

Serves: 1 hungry man
Total Fat Content Per Serving: 8 grams

Nutrition Facts

1 servings per container

Serving size	1 Omelet

Amount Per Serving

Calories	410

	% Daily Value*
Total Fat 8g	10%
Saturated Fat 1.82g	9%
Trans Fat 0g	
Cholesterol 55mg	19%
Sodium 1200mg	52%
Total Carbohydrate 36g	13%
Dietary Fiber 2g	7%
Total Sugars 4g	
Includes 0g Added Sugars	0%
Protein 44g	88%

Not a significant source of vitamin D, calcium, iron, and potassium

*The % Daily Value (DV) tells you how much a nutrient in a serving of food contributes to a daily diet. 2,000 calories a day is used for general nutrition advice.

Oatmeal Palooza

Man—where was this when I was a kid? Great for lazy Sunday mornings

1 cup Old-Fashioned Quaker Oats
1 cup skim milk
3/4 cup water
2 tablespoons firmly packed brown sugar
1/4 cup banana (chopped or sliced)
1/4 cup strawberry (chopped or sliced)
2-4 tablespoons fat-free or light whipped cream topping (I recommend the spray can kind—more fun!)

Heat milk and water in saucepan until boiling, and then stir in Quaker oats and return to boil. Reduce heat to medium and let simmer for about five minutes or until all liquid is absorbed, stirring occasionally. Remove from heat and let stand until oatmeal is at desired consistency. Mix in banana and strawberries. Top with whipped cream and eat-a-palooza!

Serves: 2
Total Fat Content Per Serving: 4.5 grams

Nutrition Facts

2 servings per container

Serving size	1 Bowl

Amount Per Serving

Calories	300

	% Daily Value*
Total Fat 4.5g	6%
Saturated Fat 1.5g	8%
Trans Fat 0g	
Cholesterol < 5mg	2%
Sodium 5mg	0%
Total Carbohydrate 55g	20%
Dietary Fiber 6g	20%
Total Sugars 26g	
Includes 0g Added Sugars	0%
Protein 10g	19%

Not a significant source of vitamin D, calcium, iron, and potassium

*The % Daily Value (DV) tells you how much a nutrient in a serving of food contributes to a daily diet. 2,000 calories a day is used for general nutrition advice.

Rhubarb Muffins

Rhubarb grows wild in my yard, so we always have lots. You can use fresh rhubarb if you can find it—or frozen will work too. Just thaw and drain if you use frozen.

1 ½ cups flour
1 teaspoon baking powder
2 teaspoons cinnamon
¼ teaspoon baking soda
¼ teaspoon salt
¼ cup egg substitute (or 2 egg whites)
1 teaspoon vanilla
2/3 cup brown sugar
2/3 cup unsweetened applesauce
1 tablespoon vegetable oil
1 cup chopped rhubarb

Preheat oven to 400 degrees. Line muffin cups with paper liners, or lightly coat with non-stick spray.

Mix together the flour, baking powder, cinnamon, baking soda and salt. In another bowl mix the egg, vanilla, brown sugar, applesauce, and oil. Then combine the dry and wet ingredients and stir until just mixed. Fold in the rhubarb.

Divide batter between 12 muffin cups and bake for 20 minutes.

Serves: 12
Total Fat Content Per Serving: 1 gram

Nutrition Facts

12 servings per container

Serving size	**1 Muffin**

Amount Per Serving

Calories 170

	% Daily Value*
Total Fat 1g	**2%**
Saturated Fat 0.17g	1%
Trans Fat 0g	
Cholesterol 0mg	**0%**
Sodium 105mg	**5%**
Total Carbohydrate 37g	**13%**
Dietary Fiber 2g	6%
Total Sugars 11g	
Includes 0g Added Sugars	0%
Protein < 1g	**1%**

Not a significant source of vitamin D, calcium, iron, and potassium

*The % Daily Value (DV) tells you how much a nutrient in a serving of food contributes to a daily diet. 2,000 calories a day is used for general nutrition advice.

Skillet-Style Breakfast

A plateful of spiced-up goodness that'll make your whole kitchen smell good. Don't be surprised if the rest of your family wants you to share!

1 large potato
1/2 cup chopped onion
1/4 cup chopped green pepper
1/4 cup chopped parsley (optional)
1 slice Jennie-O Lean Turkey Bacon
fat-free butter spray
paprika
minced garlic
seasoned black pepper

Wash the potato and poke holes in it with a fork or knife. Bake the potato for 5 minutes in a microwave oven, and let cool. Microwave a slice of Jennie-O Lean Turkey Bacon until crispy (about 5-10 seconds longer than called for in the Jennie-O instructions). Chop baked potato into bite-sized chunks and spread the chunks into a Teflon skillet that's lightly covered with fat-free, nonstick spray. Add chopped onion, chopped green pepper, and (optional) chopped parsley. Crumble bacon into the mix as well. Cover lightly with four or five pumps of fat-free butter spray. Season to taste with paprika, seasoned black pepper, and minced garlic. Cook over medium heat, stirring occasionally, until all is light brown and lightly crisped,
Serve warm on a plate or in a bowl.

Note:
For extra flavor, add a little salsa on your plate. For extra heft, top with fat-free scrambled eggs and fat-free cheese.

Serves: 1
Total Fat Content Per Serving: 3 grams

Nutrition Facts

1 servings per container

Serving size	1 Plate

Amount Per Serving

Calories	360

	% Daily Value*
Total Fat 3g	4%
Saturated Fat 0.63g	3%
Trans Fat 0g	
Cholesterol 10mg	3%
Sodium 160mg	7%
Total Carbohydrate 74g	27%
Dietary Fiber 9g	34%
Total Sugars 4g	
Includes 0g Added Sugars	0%
Protein 11g	22%

Not a significant source of vitamin D, calcium, iron, and potassium

*The % Daily Value (DV) tells you how much a nutrient in a serving of food contributes to a daily diet. 2,000 calories a day is used for general nutrition advice.

Veggie Lovers Egg-White Omelet

A hearty, home-style breakfast for any hungry man.

4 egg whites
1/4 cup chopped onion
1/4 cup chopped green pepper
1/4 cup chopped Roma tomato
black pepper
2 tablespoons Kraft Natural Shredded Fat Free Cheddar Cheese

Mix egg whites, onion, green pepper, and Roma tomatoes in a bowl until thoroughly blended. Pour egg mixture into a Teflon skillet that's lightly covered with fat-free, nonstick cooking spray and cook over medium heat. Season to taste with black pepper.

Do not stir; let the egg mixture cook until the bottom becomes firm. Then, with a plastic spatula, gently push one edge of the omelet toward the center, and do the same with the other edge. When the center seems firm, flip the entire omelet over and let it cook to desired firmness. You may want to flip the omelet one or two more times to even out the cooking, but don't let the omelet turn brown from the heat.

Fold in half and serve hot on a plate with shredded cheese sprinkled over the top.

Note: Try other veggie filling to suit your likes! Diced mushrooms, broccoli, sprouts, green onions—any veggie you like will taste good in this breakfast.

Serves: 1 hungry man
Total Fat Content Per Serving: Trace only

Nutrition Facts

1 servings per container

Serving size	1 Omelet

Amount Per Serving

Calories	140

	% Daily Value*
Total Fat 0.5g	1%
Saturated Fat 0g	0%
Trans Fat 0g	
Cholesterol < 5mg	2%
Sodium 520mg	23%
Total Carbohydrate 7g	3%
Dietary Fiber 2g	7%
Total Sugars 4g	
Includes 0g Added Sugars	0%
Protein 26g	52%

Not a significant source of vitamin D, calcium, iron, and potassium

*The % Daily Value (DV) tells you how much a nutrient in a serving of food contributes to a daily diet. 2,000 calories a day is used for general nutrition advice.

Lunch

10 low-fat choices for midday munchies

Baked Potato Soup

This one's great on cold winter days. Mmm.

3 large potatoes
1 onion, chopped
1 can skim evaporated milk
1/2 teaspoon black pepper
4 slices Jennie-O Lean Turkey Bacon
1/2 cup Kraft Natural Shredded Fat Free Cheddar Cheese
1/2 cup fat-free sour cream
salt and/or garlic salt (optional, to taste)

Cut potatoes into chunks—you can either peel the potatoes or leave the skin on, whichever you like better. Put potatoes into a saucepan, and add just enough water to cover the potatoes. Boil gently until potatoes are soft and done.
Drain off a little of the water, then add the evaporated milk and pepper. Use a potato masher to mash the potatoes slightly so that the soup is thick and chunky.

Optional: Add salt or garlic salt, seasoning to your taste. Keep the soup warm until ready to serve, but don't bring it to a boil.

When ready to serve, ladle soup into bowls and top each one with sour cream, cheese, and a slice of crumbled bacon.

Nutrition Facts	
4 servings per container	
Serving size	**1 Bowl**
Amount Per Serving	
Calories	**380**
	% Daily Value*
Total Fat 3g	**4%**
Saturated Fat 0.5g	**3%**
Trans Fat 0g	
Cholesterol 10mg	**3%**
Sodium 430mg	**19%**
Total Carbohydrate 67g	**24%**
Dietary Fiber 6g	**21%**
Total Sugars 15g	
Includes 0g Added Sugars	**0%**
Protein 20g	**40%**

Not a significant source of vitamin D, calcium, iron, and potassium

*The % Daily Value (DV) tells you how much a nutrient in a serving of food contributes to a daily diet. 2,000 calories a day is used for general nutrition advice.

Note: If you want to, before you add milk, you can also add any other vegetables you like to this soup. Broccoli, cauliflower, celery, and carrots all bring good flavor and texture. Or feel free to try something new!

Serves: 4
Total Fat Content Per Serving: 3 grams

Tip:
Consider cooking this up the night before, and then taking it to work in Tupperware the next day. Still tastes great after being warmed up in the break-room microwave! One warning though: people who smell your lunch may ask for a bite of it.

Black Bean Soup

Serve with low-fat tortilla chips and a dollop of fat-free sour cream for taste-great-ness.

1 cup finely chopped onion
2 cloves garlic, minced
2 teaspoons chili powder (or a little more if you like it spicy)
1 teaspoon ground cumin
2 cans black beans, rinsed and drained
1 can chicken broth

Spray the bottom of a large pan with cooking spray. Cook the onions and garlic over medium heat until tender. If the pan seems too dry, you can add a little water or wine to the onions and garlic as you sauté them.

When garlic and onions are tender, add the remaining ingredients. Simmer for about 15 minutes, and then serve.

If you want a thicker mixture, put about a third of the bean soup into a blender and puree for a few seconds, then return this to the rest of the soup and stir well before serving.

Serves: 4
Total Fat Content Per Serving: 1 gram

Nutrition Facts

4 servings per container

Serving size	**1 Bowl**

Amount Per Serving

Calories	**940**

	% Daily Value*
Total Fat 1g	**1%**
Saturated Fat 0g	**0%**
Trans Fat 0g	
Cholesterol 0mg	**0%**
Sodium 2370mg	**103%**
Total Carbohydrate 69g	**25%**
Dietary Fiber 1g	**4%**
Total Sugars 2g	
Includes 0g Added Sugars	**0%**
Protein 24g	**48%**

Not a significant source of vitamin D, calcium, iron, and potassium

*The % Daily Value (DV) tells you how much a nutrient in a serving of food contributes to a daily diet. 2,000 calories a day is used for general nutrition advice.

Dude, You Don't Have to be Fat

Chicken Quesadilla

I like to make this whole recipe and eat half of it fresh and hot for lunch, then save the other half for a cold, tasty snack in the afternoon.

1/2 cup diced, fully-cooked chicken breast
1 cup Kraft Natural Shredded Fat Free Mozzarella Cheese
     (or Lifetime brand of Fat Free Mozzarella Cheese, shredded)
2 tablespoons chopped green onion
2 low-fat or no-fat flour tortillas
fat-free butter spray

Spray one side of a tortilla with about four or five pumps of butter spray, and place in skillet with butter side down. Spread 1/2 cup cheese on tortilla, the spread diced chicken breast and green onion over the cheese. Top with the rest of the cheese, and the second tortilla. Spray top tortilla with about four or five pumps of butter spray.

Cook over medium heat until cheese starts to melt together, then flip over in the pan. Continue cooking, flipping occasionally, until cheese is melted and both sides are light brown. Cut in half and serve warm, or refrigerate and serve cold later.

Note: For the chicken breast, you can either grill, bake, or slow-cook it yourself, or you can use a pre-cooked version such as Tyson Grilled & Ready™ Refrigerated Fully Cooked Grilled Chicken Breast Strips.

Also, if fat-free mozzarella cheese is inexplicably hard to find in your area, substitute 1/3 cup of low-moisture, part-skim mozzarella instead. This adds 3 grams of fat to each serving, which should still be fine.

Serves: 2
Total Fat Content Per Serving: 3.5 grams

Nutrition Facts

2 servings per container

Serving size	1/2 Quesadilla

Amount Per Serving

Calories	290

	% Daily Value*
Total Fat 3.5g	4%
Saturated Fat 0g	0%
Trans Fat 0g	
Cholesterol 35mg	11%
Sodium 1130mg	49%
Total Carbohydrate 31g	11%
Dietary Fiber 3g	11%
Total Sugars 2g	
Includes 0g Added Sugars	0%
Protein 36g	72%

Not a significant source of vitamin D, calcium, iron, and potassium

*The % Daily Value (DV) tells you how much a nutrient in a serving of food contributes to a daily diet. 2,000 calories a day is used for general nutrition advice.

Chicken Salad Sandwiches

Here's good eats on a hot day. Kitchen stays cool, and your stomach gets full!

12 ounces diced, grilled chicken breast (about 2 breasts)
1/2 cup finely chopped onion (or green onion, if you prefer)
3/4 cup finely chopped cucumber
1/4 cup finely chopped grapes
1 cup fat-free mayonnaise
black pepper
8 slices low-fat, wheat bread

Mix diced chicken breast, onion, cucumber, and grapes in a bowl. Begin adding mayonnaise to the mixture, one tablespoon at a time. Add mayonnaise and stir until consistency is suitable for spreading on bread. This may be less than the 1 cup measurement—just don't use more than a cup of the mayo. Season to taste with black pepper.

Toast bread, and spread mixture on it to make a sandwich. Serve cold.

Note: For the chicken breast, you can either grill it yourself, or use a pre-cooked version such as Tyson Grilled & Ready™ Refrigerated Fully Cooked Grilled Chicken Breast Strips.

Serves: 4
Total Fat Content Per Serving: 5 grams

Nutrition Facts

4 servings per container

Serving size	**1 Sandwich**

Amount Per Serving

Calories	**340**

	% Daily Value*
Total Fat 5g	6%
Saturated Fat 0g	0%
Trans Fat 0g	
Cholesterol 50mg	17%
Sodium 1180mg	51%
Total Carbohydrate 49g	18%
Dietary Fiber 6g	21%
Total Sugars 13g	
Includes 0g Added Sugars	0%
Protein 29g	58%

Not a significant source of vitamin D, calcium, iron, and potassium

* The % Daily Value (DV) tells you how much a nutrient in a serving of food contributes to a daily diet. 2,000 calories a day is used for general nutrition advice.

Football Sandwiches

No need to wait until fall to enjoy these fist-sized beauties. Eat before, during, and after your favorite team plays on TV. Keep extras in the freezer in case everyone stops by your house to watch the big game.

1 tablespoon poppy seeds
2 tablespoons Worcestershire sauce
½ cup onion, finely diced
2 tablespoons mustard
½ cup fat-free mayonnaise
8 French rolls
48 slices of thinly sliced deli roast beef (approximately 1 pound)
16 sandwich-sized slices of fat-free cheese

Mix the poppy seeds, Worcestershire sauce, onion, mustard, and mayonnaise in a small bowl and stir until completely mixed.

Slice open the French rolls if they are not already sliced. Divide the poppy seed mixture evenly between the rolls and spread on the inside of each roll. Place two slices of cheese and six slices of roast beef inside each roll.

Close the rolls and wrap each sandwich individually in foil. Bake at 350 degrees for 20 minutes, then serve hot.

These sandwiches can be made ahead of time and kept in the freezer until you're ready to eat. If you're putting a frozen sandwich directly into the oven, bake at 350 degrees for 40 minutes.

You can also adapt this recipe with other low-fat sliced meats such as turkey, pastrami, or chicken. Just be sure you choose low-fat meats and fat-free cheese slices.

Serves: 8
Total Fat Content Per Serving: 3 grams

Nutrition Facts

8 servings per container

Serving size	1 Sandwich

Amount Per Serving

Calories	320

	% Daily Value*
Total Fat 3g	4%
Saturated Fat 1g	5%
Trans Fat 0g	
Cholesterol 40mg	13%
Sodium 1680mg	73%
Total Carbohydrate 39g	14%
Dietary Fiber 1g	4%
Total Sugars 4g	
Includes 0g Added Sugars	0%
Protein 26g	52%

Not a significant source of vitamin D, calcium, iron, and potassium

* The % Daily Value (DV) tells you how much a nutrient in a serving of food contributes to a daily diet. 2,000 calories a day is used for general nutrition advice.

French Dip Sandwiches

Amour en la bouche – Profitez!

8 French rolls
48 slices of thinly sliced deli roast beef (approximately 1 pound)
1 can (14 ounce) beef broth

Place the beef and the beef broth in a sauce pan and warm over low heat.

While the meat is warming, slice open the French rolls if they are not already sliced. Place them face up on a baking sheet, and put into an oven set on broil. Broil for a minute or two, keeping a close watch on the bread. You want it to toast evenly and not burn.

When the bread is toasted to your liking, remove from the oven.

Divide the meat evenly between the rolls, putting the tops on each roll to make a sandwich. Serve each person a small container of the remaining broth to use when dipping their sandwich.

Serves: 8
Total Fat Content Per Serving: 3 grams

Nutrition Facts

8 servings per container

Serving size — **1 Sandwich**

Amount Per Serving

Calories — **230**

	% Daily Value*
Total Fat 3g	4%
Saturated Fat 1g	5%
Trans Fat 0g	
Cholesterol 30mg	10%
Sodium 1100mg	48%
Total Carbohydrate 32g	12%
Dietary Fiber 1g	4%
Total Sugars 0g	
Includes 0g Added Sugars	0%
Protein 17g	34%

Not a significant source of vitamin D, calcium, iron, and potassium

*The % Daily Value (DV) tells you how much a nutrient in a serving of food contributes to a daily diet. 2,000 calories a day is used for general nutrition advice.

Pasta Salad

Dude, if you're gonna eat salad, at least it should taste good, right? That's where this recipe comes in. Enjoy it!

2 cups plain macaroni
2 carrots, grated
1 cup snow peas, halved
1/4 cup green onion, chopped
1/2 cup red pepper, chopped

Dressing
1/2 cup fat-free mayonnaise
1/2 cup fat-free sour cream
1 tablespoon red wine vinegar
1/2 teaspoon ground ginger
pepper (to taste)

Prepare macaroni according to directions on package. Drain macaroni and mix with vegetables. Whisk together dressing ingredients and pour over pasta and vegetables. Stir until the salad is coated with dressing. Cover and refrigerate at least two hours.

Serve cold.

Note: You can also experiment with other vegetables in this salad. For instance, try adding halved cherry tomatoes, or chopped broccoli or zucchini.

Serves: 4
Total Fat Content Per Serving: 2 grams

Nutrition Facts

4 servings per container

Serving size	1/4 Recipe

Amount Per Serving

Calories	510

	% Daily Value*
Total Fat 2g	3%
Saturated Fat 0.5g	3%
Trans Fat 0g	
Cholesterol < 5mg	2%
Sodium 260mg	11%
Total Carbohydrate 102g	37%
Dietary Fiber 6g	21%
Total Sugars 12g	
Includes 0g Added Sugars	0%
Protein 17g	34%

Not a significant source of vitamin D, calcium, iron, and potassium

*The % Daily Value (DV) tells you how much a nutrient in a serving of food contributes to a daily diet. 2,000 calories a day is used for general nutrition advice.

Shredded Chicken Barbecue Sandwiches

This one's super easy—and delicious. Cook up a batch on Sunday, and then eat it for lunch all week long.

3 boneless, skinless chicken breasts
1 ½ cups Sweet Baby Ray's Original Barbecue Sauce (or your favorite barbecue sauce)
6 low-fat, wheat hamburger buns

Trim any visible fat off the chicken breasts, and then place the breasts in a crock pot. Drench the breasts with barbecue sauce. Slow-cook on high for 3-4 hours (may take a little longer if chicken breasts are frozen), or on low for 6-8 hours.

Use two forks to shred apart the cooked meat. Stir.

If you like, add more barbecue sauce to suit your taste. Serve, either hot or cold, on a hamburger bun. Enjoy!

Serves: 6
Total Fat Content Per Serving: 3 grams

Nutrition Facts

6 servings per container

Serving size	1 Sandwich

Amount Per Serving

Calories	300

	% Daily Value*
Total Fat 3g	4%
Saturated Fat 0.5g	3%
Trans Fat 0g	
Cholesterol 35mg	12%
Sodium 800mg	35%
Total Carbohydrate 54g	20%
Dietary Fiber 1g	4%
Total Sugars 34g	
Includes 0g Added Sugars	0%
Protein 14g	28%

Not a significant source of vitamin D, calcium, iron, and potassium

* The % Daily Value (DV) tells you how much a nutrient in a serving of food contributes to a daily diet. 2,000 calories a day is used for general nutrition advice.

Dude, You Don't Have to be Fat

Stuffed Potato Palooza

This recipe is only for one potato/serving, but if you want to share with others you can simply add potatoes and stuffing, and repeat the recipe as many times as you like.

1 large potato
1/4 cup fat-free sour cream
2 tablespoons Heinz 57 Sauce (optional)
1/4 cup diced green onions
2 tablespoons Kraft Natural Shredded Fat Free Cheddar Cheese
1 slice Jennie-O Lean Turkey Bacon
black pepper

Wash the potato and poke holes in it with a fork or knife. Bake the potato for 5 minutes in a microwave oven. While potato is cooking, mix sour cream, Heinz 57 Sauce, green onion, and cheese in a bowl.

When potato is done, roll it gently on the counter to loosen the filling inside. Then slice the potato in half, and hollow out both halves while leaving the skin intact. Mash the potato filling and fold it in with the sour cream mixture. Then re-fill the potato skins with the sour cream mixture. Season with black pepper to taste.

Microwave one slice of Jennie-O Lean Turkey Bacon until crispy, and crumble the bacon over the top of the potato halves.

Serve hot and delicious!

Serves: 1
Total Fat Content Per Serving: 3

Nutrition Facts

1 servings per container

Serving size — **1 Stuffed Potato**

Amount Per Serving

Calories 450

	% Daily Value*
Total Fat 3g	4%
Saturated Fat 0.63g	3%
Trans Fat 0g	
Cholesterol 10mg	3%
Sodium 640mg	28%
Total Carbohydrate 85g	31%
Dietary Fiber 8g	29%
Total Sugars 9g	
Includes 0g Added Sugars	0%
Protein 19g	38%

Not a significant source of vitamin D, calcium, iron, and potassium

* The % Daily Value (DV) tells you how much a nutrient in a serving of food contributes to a daily diet. 2,000 calories a day is used for general nutrition advice.

Taco Burgers

Was jonesing a Taco John's taco burger one day, but didn't want 9 full grams of fat for it. So I decided to make my own low-fat version—and it tasted better anyway!

1/2 pound extra-lean (96/4) ground beef
1-3 tablespoons taco seasoning (to taste)
1 tablespoon water
1/4 cup Kraft Natural Shredded Fat Free Cheddar Cheese
1/4 cup diced tomatoes
2-4 lettuce leaves
mild taco sauce (to taste)
2 low-fat, wheat hamburger buns

Brown the beef in a skillet with water and taco seasoning (season to taste). Put 1/2 of the seasoned, cooked beef on a bun. Save the rest of the beef for a second sandwich or for future use. Add taco sauce (to taste). Top the beef as desired with cheese, diced tomatoes, and 1-2 lettuce leaves. Eat as a sandwich and enjoy!

Serves: 2
Total Fat Content Per Serving: 5 grams

Nutrition Facts

2 servings per container

Serving size	1 Taco Burger

Amount Per Serving

Calories	310

% Daily Value*

Total Fat 5g	6%
Saturated Fat 2g	10%
Trans Fat 0g	
Cholesterol 70mg	23%
Sodium 1230mg	53%
Total Carbohydrate 32g	12%
Dietary Fiber 6g	21%
Total Sugars 6g	
Includes 0g Added Sugars	0%
Protein 38g	76%

Not a significant source of vitamin D, calcium, iron, and potassium

*The % Daily Value (DV) tells you how much a nutrient in a serving of food contributes to a daily diet. 2,000 calories a day is used for general nutrition advice.

Dude, You Don't Have to be Fat

Dinner

15 delicious recipes for enjoyable evenings at home

Better-Than-Sex Lasagna

This sexy entrée is a perfect way to show off your cooking skills for your favorite girl. Serve it with a tossed salad and sourdough bread to complete the mood.

1 (26 ounce) can or jar of spaghetti sauce (choose any flavor you like that has less than 1 gram of fat per serving, such as one that uses extra garlic, veggies, or other seasonings—not one with added cheese)
1 pound extra lean ground beef
2 cups fat free cottage cheese
1/4 cup egg substitute or 2 egg whites
1/2 teaspoon dried minced garlic
2 cups fat free mozzarella cheese, shredded
        (use either Kraft or Lifetime brand of fat-free cheese)
1 box (9 ounces) no-boil lasagna

Preheat oven to 350°. Brown ground beef in a large skillet, crumbling the meat and cooking over medium heat until done. Add the spaghetti sauce and set aside.

In a separate bowl, mix the cottage cheese, egg substitute, and minced garlic. Stir well.

Spray a 9x11 or 9x13 pan with non-stick spray. Spoon about 1/2 a cup of the meat sauce into the bottom of the pan and spread around. Then put one layer of lasagna noodles over this. Cover these with about half of the remaining sauce. Put another layer of pasta over this. Spoon the cottage cheese mixture over this and spread over the pasta. Put another layer of pasta over this. Spoon the remaining sauce over the pasta and cover with the mozzarella cheese.

Bake at 350° for 45 minutes. Serve hot.

Note: If fat-free mozzarella is inexplicably hard to find in your area, substitute 1 and 1/3 cup of low-moisture, part-skim mozzarella instead. This adds 3 grams of fat to each serving, but should still be fine.

Serves: 8
Total Fat Content Per Serving: 4 grams

Nutrition Facts

8 servings per container

Serving size	1 Square

Amount Per Serving

Calories	360

	% Daily Value*
Total Fat 4g	5%
Saturated Fat 1.36g	7%
Trans Fat 0g	
Cholesterol 35mg	12%
Sodium 1450mg	63%
Total Carbohydrate 41g	15%
Dietary Fiber 4g	13%
Total Sugars 13g	
Includes 0g Added Sugars	0%
Protein 38g	76%

Not a significant source of vitamin D, calcium, iron, and potassium

*The % Daily Value (DV) tells you how much a nutrient in a serving of food contributes to a daily diet. 2,000 calories a day is used for general nutrition advice.

Chili Verde

This uses green chilies and chicken and is on the milder side. Serve with fat free sour cream and low-fat flour tortillas if you like.

1 can chicken broth
3 (4 ounce) chicken breasts
1 cup onion, diced
1 can (16 ounces) pinto beans, drained and rinsed
1 can diced green chilies
2 cloves garlic, minced
1 teaspoon cumin
1 teaspoon oregano
1/8 teaspoon ground cloves

Cut chicken into bite-sized pieces. Put all ingredients into a crock pot, and cook on low for 4 to 6 hours.

Serves: 4
Total Fat Content Per Serving: 3 grams

Nutrition Facts

4 servings per container

Serving size	1 Cup

Amount Per Serving

Calories	180

	% Daily Value*
Total Fat 3g	4%
Saturated Fat 0.62g	3%
Trans Fat 0g	
Cholesterol 50mg	16%
Sodium 660mg	29%
Total Carbohydrate 18g	7%
Dietary Fiber 6g	21%
Total Sugars 4g	
Includes 0g Added Sugars	0%
Protein 23g	46%

Not a significant source of vitamin D, calcium, iron, and potassium

* The % Daily Value (DV) tells you how much a nutrient in a serving of food contributes to a daily diet. 2,000 calories a day is used for general nutrition advice.

Chunky Chicken Stew

This is great for the winter months—hearty and filling. Serve with yeast rolls fresh from the oven.

3 small (4 ounce) boneless, skinless chicken breasts
1 cup carrots, diced
2 cups green beans (frozen beans work great)
1 cup corn (frozen corn works great too)
2 cups potatoes, peeled and diced
1 cup onion, diced
2 cloves garlic, minced
1 (15 ounce) can of tomato sauce (or V8 juice can be used if you like)
1 (16 ounce) can chicken broth
1 tablespoon Worcestershire sauce
1 teaspoon cumin

Cut the chicken into bite-sized pieces. Put all ingredients into a crock pot and cook on low for 4 to 6 hours, or until the chicken is cooked through and the vegetables are tender.

Serve hot!

Serves: 8
Total Fat Content Per Serving: 2 grams

Nutrition Facts

8 servings per container

Serving size	1 Cup

Amount Per Serving

Calories	160

	% Daily Value*
Total Fat 2g	3%
Saturated Fat 0.2g	1%
Trans Fat 0g	
Cholesterol 25mg	9%
Sodium 460mg	20%
Total Carbohydrate 25g	9%
Dietary Fiber 2g	7%
Total Sugars 4g	
Includes 0g Added Sugars	0%
Protein 11g	22%

Not a significant source of vitamin D, calcium, iron, and potassium

* The % Daily Value (DV) tells you how much a nutrient in a serving of food contributes to a daily diet. 2,000 calories a day is used for general nutrition advice.

Dude, You Don't Have to be Fat

Daddy's Home-Style Meatloaf

If you're a meat-and-potatoes kind of guy, this is for you.

2/3 cup old-fashioned oats
1/2 cup skim milk
2 tablespoons Worcestershire sauce
1 pound extra lean ground beef
1/2 cup shredded carrots
1/2 cup finely chopped onion
2 egg whites
1/2 cup reduced-fat blue cheese crumbles

Preheat oven to 350° and lightly spray a loaf pan with baking spray.

Mix the oats, milk, and Worcestershire sauce in a bowl. Let stand about 5 minutes to soften the oats. Add all of the remaining ingredients, and mix well with clean hands.

Place the meat mixture into the pan and flatten the top. Bake for 45 minutes. Cut into 8 slices.

Serves: 8
Total Fat Content Per Serving: 6 grams

Nutrition Facts

8 servings per container

Serving size	1 Slice

Amount Per Serving

Calories 150

	% Daily Value*
Total Fat 6g	7%
Saturated Fat 3g	15%
Trans Fat 0g	
Cholesterol 45mg	14%
Sodium 220mg	10%
Total Carbohydrate 8g	3%
Dietary Fiber 1g	4%
Total Sugars 3g	
Includes 0g Added Sugars	0%
Protein 19g	38%

Not a significant source of vitamin D, calcium, iron, and potassium

*The % Daily Value (DV) tells you how much a nutrient in a serving of food contributes to a daily diet. 2,000 calories a day is used for general nutrition advice.

Fancy Lad Fajitas

The title of this recipe is my shout-out to a favorite movie... but don't worry. These fajitas require no monkeys—and are a lot better than the film.

3 (4 ounce) chicken breasts
1 cup onion, diced
1 cup green or red pepper, diced
1 packet fajita seasoning mix
4 low-fat flour tortillas
fat free cheddar cheese (optional)
fat free sour cream (optional)

Lightly coat a skillet with cooking spray. Cut the chicken into narrow strips. Put chicken, onions, and pepper into skillet and cook over medium-high heat until the chicken is cooked through and the onions and peppers are tender, stirring often. Add the packet of fajita seasoning and about ½ cup of water. Continue cooking and stirring until most of the water has evaporated and the meat and vegetables are well seasoned with the fajita mix.

Serve on warm tortillas. Add fat-free cheese and fat-free sour cream if you like.

Serves: 4
Total Fat Content Per Serving: 4 grams

Nutrition Facts

4 servings per container

Serving size	1 Fajita

Amount Per Serving

Calories	230

	% Daily Value*
Total Fat 4g	5%
Saturated Fat 0.39g	2%
Trans Fat 0g	
Cholesterol 50mg	16%
Sodium 780mg	34%
Total Carbohydrate 29g	11%
Dietary Fiber 2g	7%
Total Sugars 3g	
Includes 0g Added Sugars	0%
Protein 21g	42%

Not a significant source of vitamin D, calcium, iron, and potassium

* The % Daily Value (DV) tells you how much a nutrient in a serving of food contributes to a daily diet. 2,000 calories a day is used for general nutrition advice.

Fake "Fried" Chicken Nuggets

Deep-fried chicken is like eating death on a drumstick, so I was happy when my wife discovered this more sensible, skillet-fried version of a fatty favorite from my childhood.

3 boneless, skinless chicken breasts (4 ounces each)
½ cup flour
½ teaspoon black pepper
1 tablespoon butter

Cut chicken into nugget-sized chunks (about 8 chunks per breast).

Mix flour and pepper, then dredge (roll) chicken in the flour mixture so each piece is coated. Melt butter in a frying pan and add chicken nuggets.

Cook for several minutes on medium to high heat, then turn chicken over, being careful not to let chicken burn.

Serve with your favorite fruit or vegetable side dish (such as corn or watermelon).

Serves: 4 (about 6 nuggets per serving)
Total Fat Content Per Serving: 4 grams

Nutrition Facts

4 servings per container

Serving size   **6 Nuggets**

Amount Per Serving

Calories   **220**

	% Daily Value*
Total Fat 4g	**5%**
Saturated Fat 1.75g	**9%**
Trans Fat 0g	
Cholesterol 55mg	**18%**
Sodium 210mg	**9%**
Total Carbohydrate 24g	**9%**
Dietary Fiber 0g	**0%**
Total Sugars 0g	
Includes 0g Added Sugars	**0%**
Protein 18g	**36%**

Not a significant source of vitamin D, calcium, iron, and potassium

*The % Daily Value (DV) tells you how much a nutrient in a serving of food contributes to a daily diet. 2,000 calories a day is used for general nutrition advice.

Kebaberdoodles

Getting stuff to stay on a kebob is a hassle. This recipe takes all the best stuff from a kebob and makes it easy to cook. They're great for a cook-out—you can bring your packet of food ready to toss on the grill.

3 (4-ounce) chicken breasts, cut into bite-sized cubes
2 potatoes, peeled and diced
2 cobs of corn, with husk and silk removed
1 cup of onion, diced
butter spray
garlic and herb seasoning or lemon pepper

Place four sheets of aluminum foil on your counter. On each one put ¼ of the chicken, ¼ of the potatoes, ¼ of the onion, and ½ of a cob of corn. Lightly mist with butter spray, and season with either a garlic and herb mix (like Mrs. Dash) or lemon pepper.

Wrap foil around ingredients and fold well to make a sealed packet. These can be baked in the oven (45 minutes at 350°) or placed on a grill (time will vary based on the heat on your grill, so be sure the chicken is cooked through and the potatoes are tender).

Break open a packet and enjoy!

Serves: 4
Total Fat Content Per Serving: 2.5 grams

Nutrition Facts

4 servings per container

Serving size	**1 Tinfoil Packet**

Amount Per Serving

Calories 190

	% Daily Value*
Total Fat 2.5g	3%
Saturated Fat 0.5g	3%
Trans Fat 0g	
Cholesterol 50mg	16%
Sodium 150mg	7%
Total Carbohydrate 25g	9%
Dietary Fiber 3g	11%
Total Sugars 4g	
Includes 0g Added Sugars	0%
Protein 20g	40%

Not a significant source of vitamin D, calcium, iron, and potassium

*The % Daily Value (DV) tells you how much a nutrient in a serving of food contributes to a daily diet. 2,000 calories a day is used for general nutrition advice.

Parmesan Pasta with Chicken

This is a quick and easy meal—and really tasty.

2 small (4-ounce) chicken breasts
8 ounces uncooked spaghetti (recommend wheat or multi-grain pasta)
butter spray
seasonings

Grill chicken, adding any seasonings you like such as minced garlic, crushed oregano, or other dried herbs. When chicken is cooked through, remove from grill and cut into bite-sized pieces.

While chicken is grilling, cook the pasta according to directions on packaging. Drain and place in serving dish. Spray with 10 pumps of the butter spray. Sprinkle lightly with additional herbs such as garlic powder or Italian seasoning. Add the chicken, toss, and serve.

Serves: 4
Total Fat Content Per Serving: 1 gram

Nutrition Facts

4 servings per container

Serving size	1/4 Recipe

Amount Per Serving

Calories 150

	% Daily Value*
Total Fat 1g	1%
Saturated Fat 0.2g	1%
Trans Fat 0g	
Cholesterol 35mg	11%
Sodium 50mg	2%
Total Carbohydrate 17g	6%
Dietary Fiber 2g	7%
Total Sugars 1g	
Includes 0g Added Sugars	0%
Protein 16g	32%

Not a significant source of vitamin D, calcium, iron, and potassium

* The % Daily Value (DV) tells you how much a nutrient in a serving of food contributes to a daily diet. 2,000 calories a day is used for general nutrition advice.

Pseudo Big Mac

A real Big Mac is packed with fat. Make your own at home and enjoy the power without the pudge.

The Not-So-Secret-Sauce:
½ cup fat free mayo
2 tablespoons fat-free French dressing
4 teaspoons sweet relish
1 tablespoon dried onion flakes
1 teaspoon white vinegar
1 teaspoon sugar

The Burgers
1 pound extra lean ground beef
4 lettuce leaves
4 slices of fat free American cheese
8 dill pickle slices
4 slices of onion
4 wheat hamburger buns (look for buns that have 1 to 1.5 grams of fat per bun)

For the sauce, mix all the ingredients in a small bowl and set aside for about 15 minutes so the onion flakes soften.

Divide beef into four equal pieces, and form into patties. Grill, broil, or pan fray (with no added oil) depending on your preference. Then assemble the burgers so you have one patty, 1/4 of the sauce, lettuce, cheese, pickles, onion, and the bun.

Serves: 4
Total Fat Content Per Serving: 6 grams

Nutrition Facts

4 servings per container

Serving size	1 Sandwich

Amount Per Serving

Calories 290

	% Daily Value*
Total Fat 6g	7%
Saturated Fat 2g	10%
Trans Fat 0g	
Cholesterol 70mg	23%
Sodium 1000mg	43%
Total Carbohydrate 28g	10%
Dietary Fiber 6g	21%
Total Sugars 9g	
Includes 0g Added Sugars	0%
Protein 33g	66%

Not a significant source of vitamin D, calcium, iron, and potassium

*The % Daily Value (DV) tells you how much a nutrient in a serving of food contributes to a daily diet. 2,000 calories a day is used for general nutrition advice.

Southwest Chili

This meal is hearty and about the easiest recipe you'll find.
Make it spicier by choosing a hotter salsa.

1 pound extra lean ground beef
1 jar of your favorite salsa
1 can of black beans, rinsed
1 (10 ounce) bag of frozen corn

Put all ingredients into a crock pot. Cook on low for 2 hours, then stir well to break up the ground beef. Cook another 2 hours before serving. Stir again, making sure all the meat is crumbled. Can be served with fat free sour cream or fat free cheese if you like.

Serves: 8
Total Fat Content Per Serving: 2.5 grams

Nutrition Facts

8 servings per container

Serving size	1 Bowl

Amount Per Serving

Calories 150

	% Daily Value*
Total Fat 2.5g	**3%**
Saturated Fat 0.75g	**4%**
Trans Fat 0g	
Cholesterol 35mg	**11%**
Sodium 640mg	**28%**
Total Carbohydrate 19g	**7%**
Dietary Fiber 3g	**11%**
Total Sugars 2g	
Includes 0g Added Sugars	**0%**
Protein 16g	**32%**

Not a significant source of vitamin D, calcium, iron, and potassium

*The % Daily Value (DV) tells you how much a nutrient in a serving of food contributes to a daily diet. 2,000 calories a day is used for general nutrition advice.

Stir-Fry Extravaganza

Lots of veggies and flavor. Niice.

4 small (4 ounce) chicken breasts, cut into strips
1 cup onion, diced
1 cup red or green pepper, diced
2 cups sugar snap peas
1 cup carrots, thinly sliced
3 cloves garlic, minced
3 tablespoons soy sauce
2 cups rice, prepared

Lightly coat skillet with cooking spray. Heat skillet and then add the chicken. Cook, stirring constantly, until chicken begins to lose its pink color.

Add all the veggies and the garlic, and continue to cook, stirring constantly. If mixture seems like it is sticking to the pan, add a small amount of water (carefully though—avoid splattering!). Cook until the chicken is done and the veggies are at your preferred tenderness (some like them a bit crunchy, while others prefer very soft).

Add the soy sauce and stir well.

Serve over rice. You can also add more soy sauce to taste.

Serves: 8
Total Fat Content Per Serving: 1.5 grams

Nutrition Facts

8 servings per container

Serving size	1 Cup

Amount Per Serving

Calories 140

	% Daily Value*
Total Fat 1.5g	**2%**
Saturated Fat 0.26g	**1%**
Trans Fat 0g	
Cholesterol 35mg	**11%**
Sodium 500mg	**22%**
Total Carbohydrate 17g	**6%**
Dietary Fiber 2g	**7%**
Total Sugars 3g	
Includes 0g Added Sugars	**0%**
Protein 15g	**30%**

Not a significant source of vitamin D, calcium, iron, and potassium

*The % Daily Value (DV) tells you how much a nutrient in a serving of food contributes to a daily diet. 2,000 calories a day is used for general nutrition advice.

Stuffed Pizza Pies

One of my favorites! Hope you like it as much as I do.

1/2 Amy's Delicious Dinner Rolls Recipe (see page 206)
1 can (26 oz) Hunt's Garlic & Herb Spaghetti Sauce
1 3/4 cups Kraft Natural Shredded Fat Free Mozzarella Cheese
        (or Lifetime brand of Fat Free Mozzarella Cheese, shredded)
32 slices Hormel Turkey Pepperoni
1 pound extra lean ground beef (96% fat free) (optional)
1 green pepper, chopped (optional)
Pineapple chunks (optional)
Onion, chopped (optional)

Make 1/2 of "Amy's Delicious Dinner Rolls Recipe" dough and set it aside.

If you're using the ground beef filling, go ahead and brown the ground beef now as well, and set it aside.

Preheat your oven to 350 degrees.

Divide the dinner roll dough into 8 balls of equal size. Place one on a floured surface and use a rolling pin to roll dough into a circle about the size of a man's outstretched fingers.

Place a spoonful of spaghetti sauce on the spread-out dough, and add a layer of shredded mozzarella cheese. Then add a sampling of any or all of the pizza toppings to the center of the dough (such as a spoonful of ground beef, three or four pepperoni slices, chopped green peppers, and so on).

Be careful not to overfill the dough with toppings, as you don't want anything to burst out when the stuffed pizza pie is sealed.

(continued next page)

Nutrition Facts

8 servings per container

Serving size	1 Pizza Pie, All Toppings

Amount Per Serving

Calories	**560**

	% Daily Value*
Total Fat 4.5g	**6%**
Saturated Fat 1.38g	**7%**
Trans Fat 0g	
Cholesterol 40mg	**14%**
Sodium 1760mg	**76%**
Total Carbohydrate 93g	**34%**
Dietary Fiber 3g	**11%**
Total Sugars 15g	
Includes 0g Added Sugars	**0%**
Protein 28g	**56%**

Not a significant source of vitamin D, calcium, iron, and potassium

* The % Daily Value (DV) tells you how much a nutrient in a serving of food contributes to a daily diet. 2,000 calories a

Fold the dough until the edges meet, and then pinch the edges together securely so no filling shows. It's important that the dough for these pies be sealed completely, as the sauce will seep out during cooking.

Repeat the process to make additional stuffed pizza pies until all the dough and the filling have been used (8 meat pies total). You will have extra sauce left over—set this aside.

Place the stuffed pizza pies on a cooking sheet that's been lightly coated with cooking spray, and bake at 350 degrees for about 15 or 20 minutes or until dough is lightly browned. Serve hot with the remaining sauce for dipping.

Note: If fat-free mozzarella is inexplicably hard to find in your area, substitute 2/3 cup of low-moisture, part-skim mozzarella instead. This adds 1.5 grams of fat to each serving, which should still be fine.

Serves: 8
Total Fat Content Per Serving:
• Pepperoni only: 3 grams
• Beef only: 4 grams
• Pepperoni & beef: 5 grams
• Green pepper, and/or onion, and/or pineapple: 2 grams;
• All toppings: 4.5 grams

Dude, You Don't Have to be Fat

Super Spaghetti

Hearty, classic Italian dish with added veggies. This one's always a hit when guests come over for dinner.

1 (26 ounce) can of Hunt's Garlic & Herb Pasta Sauce (or another tomato-based pasta sauce)
1 pound extra lean ground beef
12 ounces of spaghetti (recommend multigrain pasta)
½ cup green pepper, diced
½ cup onion, diced
2 cloves garlic, minced
¼ cup reduced-fat Parmesan cheese

Note: You can also add ½ cup of any of these veggies (diced or shredded) for added flavor and nutrition. Add as many veggies as you like!
* zucchini
* mushrooms
* carrots
* red peppers
* tomatoes
* celery
* eggplant

Brown the ground beef, then add the onion, green pepper, and garlic. Cook until the veggies are tender. Add the sauce and the Parmesan cheese and simmer until ready to serve.

Cook the pasta according to the direction on packaging. Drain, and serve with the spaghetti sauce.

Serves: 6
Total Fat Content Per Serving: 6 grams

Nutrition Facts

6 servings per container

Serving size	1/6 Recipe

Amount Per Serving

Calories **380**

	% Daily Value*
Total Fat 6g	8%
Saturated Fat 1.96g	10%
Trans Fat 0g	
Cholesterol 45mg	14%
Sodium 820mg	36%
Total Carbohydrate 53g	19%
Dietary Fiber 8g	27%
Total Sugars 7g	
Includes 0g Added Sugars	0%
Protein 30g	60%

Not a significant source of vitamin D, calcium, iron, and potassium

*The % Daily Value (DV) tells you how much a nutrient in a serving of food contributes to a daily diet. 2,000 calories a day is used for general nutrition advice.

Tilapia Tacos

If you like fish tacos, this is the meal for you!.

1 teaspoon cumin
1/8 teaspoon black pepper
2 (6-ounce) tilapia fillets
1/3 cup fat-free mayo
Zest and juice of ½ a lime
2 tablespoons fresh cilantro, chopped
1 teaspoon chili powder
8 (6-inch) corn tortillas
1 cup romaine lettuce, chopped
1 large tomato, chopped

Preheat oven to 450°.

Mix the cumin and pepper, then sprinkle over the tilapia fillets. Place the fish, with the skin down, in a baking dish that you've lightly sprayed with non-stick spray.

Cover with foil and bake 10 minutes. When fish is done, cut into strips.

In a clean bowl mix the mayo, lime zest and juice, cilantro, and chili powder.

Warm the tortillas.

On each tortilla place fish, lettuce, tomato, and a dollop of the flavored mayo. Serve to applause.

Serves: 4 (two tacos per serving)
Total Fat Content Per Serving: 4 grams

Nutrition Facts

4 servings per container

Serving size	2 Tacos

Amount Per Serving

Calories	220

	% Daily Value*
Total Fat 4g	5%
Saturated Fat 0.78g	4%
Trans Fat 0g	
Cholesterol 0mg	0%
Sodium 310mg	13%
Total Carbohydrate 29g	11%
Dietary Fiber 4g	14%
Total Sugars 4g	
Includes 0g Added Sugars	0%
Protein 19g	38%

Not a significant source of vitamin D, calcium, iron, and potassium

*The % Daily Value (DV) tells you how much a nutrient in a serving of food contributes to a daily diet. 2,000 calories a day is used for general nutrition advice.

Zesty Lemon Salmon

Lemon, herbs, and salmon … eat and enjoy.

1 cup bread crumbs
Zest and juice of ½ a lemon
½ teaspoon oregano
¼ cup fat-free mayonnaise
2 teaspoons Dijon mustard
4 (5-ounce) salmon fillets
Black pepper

Preheat oven to 400°.

Mix bread crumbs, lemon zest, and oregano together. In another bowl mix the mayo, mustard, and lemon juice.

Place the salmon in a baking dish that you've lightly coated with non-stick spray. Brush the mayo mixture on each fillet. Sprinkle the bread crumb mixture over the top, and add pepper if you like. Lightly spray with butter spray, just one pump per fillet.

Bake 10-15 minutes or until crumbs are lightly brown.

Serves: 4
Total Fat Content Per Serving: 9 grams

Nutrition Facts

4 servings per container

Serving size	1 5 oz. Filet

Amount Per Serving

Calories	300

	% Daily Value*
Total Fat 9g	12%
Saturated Fat 1.67g	8%
Trans Fat 0g	
Cholesterol 80mg	26%
Sodium 410mg	18%
Total Carbohydrate 20g	7%
Dietary Fiber 2g	7%
Total Sugars 3g	
Includes 0g Added Sugars	0%
Protein 28g	56%

Not a significant source of vitamin D, calcium, iron, and potassium

* The % Daily Value (DV) tells you how much a nutrient in a serving of food contributes to a daily diet. 2,000 calories a day is used for general nutrition advice.

Desserts

10 sweet treats for after-meal delight

Baked Apple Crisp
(with Whipped Cream Topping)

Hard to imagine Christmastime without this tasty treat near-by. And don't tell your kids, but this is also delicious served cold, for breakfast.

For the apple base:
5 cups of apples, peeled and either diced or sliced
2 tablespoons flour
1/2 cup sugar
2 teaspoons cinnamon
1/2 cup water

For the topping:
3/4 cup quick-cooking oats (not cooked yet though!)
3/4 cup brown sugar
1/4 teaspoon baking powder
3/4 cup flour
1/4 teaspoon baking soda
1/3 cup fat-free vanilla yogurt
fat-free or light whipped cream topping (I recommend the spray can kind—more fun!)

Mix together the ingredients for the apple base, and spread out in a 9x13 pan. Set aside the whipped cream for later use.

In a separate bowl, prepare the topping by mixing the rest of the topping ingredients together, adding the vanilla yogurt last. It should be a crumbly, gooey mixture (it'll firm up during baking). Spread the topping mixture over the top of the apple base.

Bake at 350 for 35 minutes. Serve hot with fat-free whipped cream on top!

Serves: 8
Total Fat Content Per Serving: 2 grams

Nutrition Facts

8 servings per container

Serving size	1/8 Recipe

Amount Per Serving

Calories	260

	% Daily Value*
Total Fat 2g	3%
Saturated Fat 1.19g	6%
Trans Fat 0g	
Cholesterol < 5mg	2%
Sodium 45mg	2%
Total Carbohydrate 38g	14%
Dietary Fiber 1g	4%
Total Sugars 21g	
Includes 0g Added Sugars	0%
Protein 2g	5%

Not a significant source of vitamin D, calcium, iron, and potassium

* The % Daily Value (DV) tells you how much a nutrient in a serving of food contributes to a daily diet. 2,000 calories a day is used for general nutrition advice.

Banana Cream Pie

No worries about heating up your kitchen with this cool treat.

1 reduced-fat graham cracker crust
2 medium bananas
2½ cups fat-free milk
2 small boxes of instant banana-flavored pudding mix
1 container (8 ounce) fat-free whipped topping

Slice the bananas and place the slices on the bottom of the prepared graham cracker crust. Set aside.

In a bowl, stir together the milk and both boxes of pudding mix. Use a whisk to mix thoroughly so there are no lumps. Beat for about 2 minutes. Pour this mixture over the banana slices and put the pie into the refrigerator to set. After about 2 hours, remove from the refrigerator and gently spoon the whipped topping over the pie.

Smooth the topping so it covers the entire pie. Serve cold.

Serves: 8
Total Fat Content Per Serving: 3.5 grams

Nutrition Facts

8 servings per container

Serving size	1 Slice

Amount Per Serving

Calories	260

	% Daily Value*
Total Fat 3.5g	4%
Saturated Fat 1g	5%
Trans Fat 0g	
Cholesterol 0mg	0%
Sodium 510mg	22%
Total Carbohydrate 52g	19%
Dietary Fiber 1g	4%
Total Sugars 34g	
Includes 0g Added Sugars	0%
Protein 4g	8%

Not a significant source of vitamin D, calcium, iron, and potassium

*The % Daily Value (DV) tells you how much a nutrient in a serving of food contributes to a daily diet. 2,000 calories a day is used for general nutrition advice.

Bon Bon Cookies

These little bites are sweet and have a surprise in each one!

½ cup fat-free vanilla yogurt
1 tablespoon vanilla extract
¾ cup powdered sugar
1 ½ cups flour
1/8 teaspoon salt
¼ cup milk chocolate chips

For the glaze
1 cup powdered sugar
1 tablespoon fat-free milk
1 teaspoon vanilla or almond extract

Mix the yogurt and vanilla extract together. Then work in the powdered sugar and flour until dough holds together well. You may need to add a bit more flour if the dough is too sticky. For each cookie, take about a tablespoon of dough into your hand and press 3 to 4 chocolate chips into the center. Fold the dough around the chips so they are in the center of the ball. Place balls about an inch apart on a baking pan that you've lightly coated with cooking spray.

Bake at 350 degrees for about 15 minutes. Cookies will not be brown, but they will be firm. Allow to cool.

For the glaze: Beat powdered sugar, milk, and extract together until smooth. If mixture is too thick, add a teaspoon of milk. If you like, add a few drops of food coloring to the glaze. Next, dip the top of each cookie into the glaze and allow glaze to set for about one hour. You can also add sprinkles, colored sugar, or coconut to each cookie immediately after dipping in the glaze. And of course you can try different treats inside the cookies such as semi-sweet or butterscotch chips, jelly, or tiny bits of dried fruit.

Makes about 24 cookies.
Total Fat Content Per Serving (2 cookies): 1 gram

Nutrition Facts	
12 servings per container	
Serving size	**2 Cookies**

Amount Per Serving	
Calories	**210**

	% Daily Value*
Total Fat 1g	**1%**
Saturated Fat 0.83g	**4%**
Trans Fat 0g	
Cholesterol < 5mg	**1%**
Sodium 30mg	**1%**
Total Carbohydrate 44g	**16%**
Dietary Fiber 0g	**0%**
Total Sugars 20g	
Includes 0g Added Sugars	**0%**
Protein 0g	**1%**

Not a significant source of vitamin D, calcium, iron, and potassium

*The % Daily Value (DV) tells you how much a nutrient in a serving of food contributes to a daily diet. 2,000 calories a day is used for general nutrition advice.

Chocolate Lava Cake

This cake is a bit unusual in that you make it in a crock pot. It's super gooey and best served hot. Delicious!

1 ¾ cups brown sugar, divided
1 cup flour
½ cup unsweetened cocoa, divided
1 ½ teaspoons baking powder
½ teaspoon salt
½ cup skim milk
1 tablespoon melted butter
½ teaspoon vanilla
1 ¾ cup boiling water

Mix 1 cup of the brown sugar, ¼ cup of the cocoa, and all of the flour, baking powder, and salt. Stir the milk, butter, and vanilla together in a separate bowl, then add this to the dry mixture.

Pour this thick batter into a crock pot that you've lightly coated with cooking spray.

In a clean bowl, mix the remaining brown sugar and cocoa. Sprinkle this over the batter, but do not stir. Pour the boiling water over this entire mixture.

Again, do not stir!

Cover and cook on high for 90 minutes.

Serves: 8
Total Fat Content Per Serving: 2 grams

Nutrition Facts

8 servings per container

Serving size	1/8 Recipe

Amount Per Serving

Calories	330

	% Daily Value*
Total Fat 2g	3%
Saturated Fat 0.88g	4%
Trans Fat 0g	
Cholesterol < 5mg	1%
Sodium 310mg	13%
Total Carbohydrate 70g	25%
Dietary Fiber 2g	7%
Total Sugars 43g	
Includes 0g Added Sugars	0%
Protein < 1g	1%

Not a significant source of vitamin D, calcium, iron, and potassium

* The % Daily Value (DV) tells you how much a nutrient in a serving of food contributes to a daily diet. 2,000 calories a day is used for general nutrition advice.

Cupcake Heaven

Easy to make and tasty to eat—you CAN have your cake and eat it too!

1 dry cake mix, any flavor
¾ cup egg substitute (such as Egg Beaters)
1/3 cup apple sauce
water as directed on cake mix

For the glaze
1 cup powdered sugar
¼ teaspoon vanilla extract
1 tablespoon fat-free milk

Place cupcake liners in cupcake tin, or lightly spray the cups with non-stick spray, and set aside.

Dump the cake mix into a bowl, and add egg substitute, apple sauce, and the amount of water listed on the cake mix box. Beat for about 2 minutes or until the batter is smooth.

Pour batter into the prepared cupcake pans and bake at 350 degrees for 20 minutes.

Cool thoroughly.

To make the icing, stir together powdered sugar, vanilla extract, and milk until smooth. Drizzle over each cupcake, then let icing set for at least 1 hour before serving.

Serves: 24
Total Fat Content Per Serving: 1 grams

Nutrition Facts

24 servings per container

Serving size	**1 Cupcake**

Amount Per Serving

Calories	**110**

	% Daily Value*
Total Fat 1g	**1%**
Saturated Fat 0.5g	**3%**
Trans Fat 0g	
Cholesterol 0mg	**0%**
Sodium 150mg	**7%**
Total Carbohydrate 24g	**9%**
Dietary Fiber 0g	**0%**
Total Sugars 15g	
Includes 0g Added Sugars	**0%**
Protein 2g	**4%**

Not a significant source of vitamin D, calcium, iron, and potassium

*The % Daily Value (DV) tells you how much a nutrient in a serving of food contributes to a daily diet. 2,000 calories a day is used for general nutrition advice.

Dad's Delicious Divinity

This candy is so airy and light—it's like eating clouds!

2 ½ cups sugar
½ cup light corn syrup
2 egg whites
1 teaspoon vanilla
¼ teaspoon salt
½ cup water

In a heavy pan mix the sugar, corn syrup, water, and salt. Cook and stir over medium heat. Keep cooking and stirring until the mixture comes to a boil. Then stop stirring and let it boil gently. While this is cooking, beat the egg whites to stiff peaks.

When the boiling mixture reaches 250 degrees, remove it from the heat and begin pouring a thin stream of the hot syrup over the egg whites, beating constantly. (This is when it's handy to have someone help you. You can do the beating while someone else pours the stream of syrup. Or get a fancy mixer on a stand so you can keep your hands free.)

Keep pouring and beating at high speed until all the syrup is mixed in. Add the vanilla, and continue beating for 4 to 5 more minutes or until the mixture begins to hold its shape. Drop dollops of the stiff mixture onto waxed paper, or spread it into a 10x6x2 pan that you've lightly coated with baking spray. Cool.

If you used the pan, cut candy into squares. Eat. Save some for a friend, if you like your friend. Otherwise don't worry about it.

Serves: about 36 pieces
Total Fat Content Per Serving: 0 grams

Tip:
Be sure you have an electric mixer that's sturdy when you make this candy—it requires a lot of beating. You'll need a candy thermometer too. Yes, go buy one.

Nutrition Facts

36 servings per container

Serving size	1 piece

Amount Per Serving

Calories	50

% Daily Value*

Total Fat 0g	0%
Saturated Fat 0g	0%
Trans Fat 0g	
Cholesterol 0mg	0%
Sodium 25mg	1%
Total Carbohydrate 5g	2%
Dietary Fiber 0g	0%
Total Sugars 2g	
Includes 0g Added Sugars	0%
Protein 0g	0%

Not a significant source of vitamin D, calcium, iron, and potassium

* The % Daily Value (DV) tells you how much a nutrient in a serving of food contributes to a daily diet. 2,000 calories a day is used for general nutrition advice.

Lucky Lemon Cheesecake

Let's just say that whenever we make this at my house, good things happen. 'Nuff said.

2 (8 ounce) packages of fat free cream cheese
¼ cup low-fat graham cracker crumbs
1 (14 ounce) can sweetened condensed milk
4 egg whites
¼ cup egg substitute such as Egg Beaters
1/3 cup lemon juice
1/ teaspoon vanilla
¼ cup flour

You may need to make your own graham cracker crumbs. Crush a few low-fat graham crackers with a rolling pin to make the crumbs.

Preheat oven to 300 degrees. Spray the bottom of an 8-inch spring-form pan with cooking spray. Sprinkle the graham cracker crumbs on the bottom of the pan. Use a mixer to beat the cream cheese until it's light and fluffy. Beat in the sweetened condensed milk, then blend in the egg whites, the egg substitute, the lemon juice, and the vanilla. Then use a spoon to stir the flour in.

Pour this mixture over the graham cracker crumbs. Bake for 45 minutes or until the center springs back when touched. Cool for about an hour, then place in the refrigerator.

If you like, serve with fresh fruit.

Serves: 10
Total Fat Content Per Serving (1 slice): trace amounts only

Nutrition Facts

10 servings per container

Serving size	1 Slice

Amount Per Serving

Calories	260

	% Daily Value*
Total Fat 0.5g	1%
Saturated Fat 0g	0%
Trans Fat 0g	
Cholesterol 15mg	5%
Sodium 450mg	19%
Total Carbohydrate 46g	17%
Dietary Fiber 0g	0%
Total Sugars 37g	
Includes 0g Added Sugars	0%
Protein 13g	26%

Not a significant source of vitamin D, calcium, iron, and potassium

* The % Daily Value (DV) tells you how much a nutrient in a serving of food contributes to a daily diet. 2,000 calories a day is used for general nutrition advice.

Patriotic Parfait

Eating fruit has never felt more statesmanlike!

2 cup sliced strawberries
2 cups blueberries
1 small container (8 ounces) fat-free whipped topping

For each parfait, put ¼ cup of strawberries in the bottom of a clear cup or glass. Add a dollop of the whipped topping. Layer ½ cup of blueberries on top of this, and top off with the another dollop of whipped topping.

Serves: 4
Total Fat Content Per Serving: less than 1 gram

Nutrition Facts

4 servings per container

Serving size	1 Cup

Amount Per Serving

Calories	140

	% Daily Value*
Total Fat 1g	1%
Saturated Fat 0g	0%
Trans Fat 0g	
Cholesterol 0mg	0%
Sodium 10mg	0%
Total Carbohydrate 33g	12%
Dietary Fiber 5g	18%
Total Sugars 6g	
Includes 0g Added Sugars	0%
Protein < 1g	1%

Not a significant source of vitamin D, calcium, iron, and potassium

* The % Daily Value (DV) tells you how much a nutrient in a serving of food contributes to a daily diet. 2,000 calories a day is used for general nutrition advice.

Dude, You Don't Have to be Fat

Soft Molasses Drop Cookies

An old family recipe handed down by my wife's grandmother—and adapted to get the most "fridge benefits" out of it. But be careful, though, these cookies are addictive.

1/4 cup applesauce
1/2 cup molasses
1/2 cup skim milk
1 teaspoon vinegar
1/2 cup sugar
2 teaspoons baking soda
2 1/2 cups flour
1 teaspoon ginger
1 teaspoon cinnamon
1/4 teaspoon nutmeg
1/2 teaspoon salt

First, mix the wet ingredients in one bowl, and the dry ingredients in another bowl. Then combine all ingredients and beat together until it forms well-mixed dough. Spoon portions of the dough onto cookie sheets lightly coated with non-stick cooking spray. Preheat the oven to 350 degrees as you do this.

Bake cookies at 350 degrees for 8 to 10 minutes, then cool on a rack. Serve at room temperature.

Yield: about 48 cookies
Total Fat Content Per Cookie: Trace only

Nutrition Facts

48 servings per container

Serving size	1 Cookie

Amount Per Serving

Calories 40

	% Daily Value*
Total Fat 0g	0%
Saturated Fat 0g	0%
Trans Fat 0g	
Cholesterol 0mg	0%
Sodium 80mg	3%
Total Carbohydrate 8g	3%
Dietary Fiber 0g	0%
Total Sugars 2g	
Includes 0g Added Sugars	0%
Protein < 1g	1%

Not a significant source of vitamin D, calcium, iron, and potassium

*The % Daily Value (DV) tells you how much a nutrient in a serving of food contributes to a daily diet. 2,000 calories a day is used for general nutrition advice.

Sweet Lemonade Pie

This is a super-easy, no-bake pie my mama used to make for my birthdays. Cool and light, it's perfect for a family get-together during the holidays.

1 can fat-free sweetened condensed milk
1 can (6 ounce) frozen lemonade concentrate
1 container (8 ounce) fat-free non-dairy whipped topping (i.e. Cool Whip)
1 reduced-fat prepared graham cracker pie crust

Gently stir the sweetened condensed milk and lemonade concentrate together, then fold in the Cool Whip. Spoon mixture into pie shell. Refrigerate for two hours, then serve cold.

Note: This pie is also good with fruit toppings spread on the top, such as fat-free cherry pie filling, or sliced strawberries, kiwi slices, and more.

Serves: 8
Total Fat Content Per Serving: 3.5 grams

Nutrition Facts

8 servings per container

Serving size	1 Slice

Amount Per Serving

Calories	260

	% Daily Value*
Total Fat 3.5g	4%
Saturated Fat 1g	5%
Trans Fat 0g	
Cholesterol 0mg	0%
Sodium 170mg	7%
Total Carbohydrate 51g	19%
Dietary Fiber 1g	4%
Total Sugars 40g	
Includes 0g Added Sugars	0%
Protein 5g	10%

Not a significant source of vitamin D, calcium, iron, and potassium

* The % Daily Value (DV) tells you how much a nutrient in a serving of food contributes to a daily diet. 2,000 calories a day is used for general nutrition advice.

Snacks & Sides
10 tasty recipes for anytime eatin'!

Amy's Delicious Dinner Rolls

This versatile recipe makes a great side dish with just about any entrée, and these rolls are also an excellent on-the-go snack for pretty much anywhere and anytime.

5 to 6 cups flour
1 tablespoon active dry yeast (or one packet)
2 cups skim milk
2 tablespoons sugar
1 tablespoon vegetable oil
2 teaspoons salt

In a large bowl stir together 2 cup of the flour, the yeast, the sugar, and the salt. Set aside. In a saucepan heat the milk and oil together to 120 degrees. Add this to the flour mixture and beat with an electric mixer for 3 minutes. Then gradually begin adding in more flour, beating constantly, until this becomes too thick to manage.

Remove the mixer and stir in more flour by hand. Stir in as much as you can, then turn the dough onto a lightly floured counter and knead. Knead and add more flour until the dough is smooth and elastic. This will take about 5 minutes. Shape the dough into a ball, and place into a bowl that you've lightly coated with baking spray. Cover and let rise in a warm place for about 1 hour.

Punch down the dough. Cover again and let rest for about 10 minutes. Then divide into 12 balls. Place these into a 9x13 pan you've lightly coated with baking spray. Cover and let rise for 30 minutes.
Bake at 375 degrees for 12-15 minutes or until the tops of the rolls are golden brown.

Note: Feel free to add a little lunchmeat and mustard for a hunger-beating snack-sandwich in the mid-afternoon or evening. Or slather on your favorite jelly for a sweet snack in the morning. Cut these into bite-sized chunks and they're also good for dipping into fat-free cheese dips or other low-fat sauces.

Serves 12.
Total Fat Content Per Serving: 1 gram

Nutrition Facts

12 servings per container

Serving size	**1 Roll**

Amount Per Serving

Calories	**220**

	% Daily Value*
Total Fat 1g	**1%**
Saturated Fat 0.17g	**1%**
Trans Fat 0g	
Cholesterol 0mg	**0%**
Sodium 510mg	**22%**
Total Carbohydrate 46g	**17%**
Dietary Fiber 2g	**7%**
Total Sugars 4g	
Includes 0g Added Sugars	**0%**
Protein 7g	**14%**

Not a significant source of vitamin D, calcium, iron, and potassium

*The % Daily Value (DV) tells you how much a nutrient in a serving of food contributes to a daily diet. 2,000 calories a day is used for general nutrition advice.

Dude, You Don't Have to be Fat

Bac-el
(pronounced "BAKE-el")

Hey, I just had me one o' these right now! Great for a quick-n-easy mid-afternoon snack.

1 Lender's Onion Bagel
1 slice Jennie-O Lean Turkey Bacon
Fat-free cream cheese (spread to taste)

Toast the bagel. Cook the bacon in a microwave.
Spread fat-free cream cheese on both sides of the bagel, then tear the bacon strip in half and place it in the cream cheese on of one side of the bagel. Cover everything with the other side of the bagel, and each as a sandwich.

Serves: 1
Total Fat Content Per Serving: 4 grams

Nutrition Facts

1 servings per container

Serving size   **1 Bagel Sandwich**

Amount Per Serving

Calories   300

	% Daily Value*
Total Fat 4g	**5%**
Saturated Fat 0.5g	3%
Trans Fat 0g	
Cholesterol 20mg	**7%**
Sodium 880mg	**38%**
Total Carbohydrate 43g	**16%**
Dietary Fiber 2g	7%
Total Sugars 4g	
Includes 0g Added Sugars	0%
Protein 17g	**34%**

Not a significant source of vitamin D, calcium, iron, and potassium

*The % Daily Value (DV) tells you how much a nutrient in a serving of food contributes to a daily diet. 2,000 calories a day is used for general nutrition advice.

Bestest Banana Bread Ever

Another fantastic family recipe, adapted for the Dude, You Don't Have to be Fat man. Nobody will believe you when you tell 'em it's fat free….

2 cups flour
1 cup sugar
1/2 cup fat-free cream cheese
4 egg whites
3 tablespoons fat-free sour cream
3 large bananas
1 teaspoon vanilla extract
1 teaspoon salt
1 teaspoon baking soda

Mix sugar and cream cheese until smooth. Add in everything else, except flour, and beat well. Add flour last. Pour into bread loaf pan that's lightly coated with fat-free, non-stick spray, and bake at 350 for one hour.

Makes one large loaf (about 8 slices).

Note: Most everyone in my family likes this with a ¼ cup of chocolate chips added to the batter before cooking.

Serves: 8 slices
Total Fat Content Per Serving (1 slice): Without chocolate chips, 0 grams; With chocolate chips, 2 grams

Nutrition Facts

8 servings per container

Serving size	1 Slice

Amount Per Serving

Calories	250

	% Daily Value*
Total Fat 0g	0%
Saturated Fat 0g	0%
Trans Fat 0g	
Cholesterol < 5mg	1%
Sodium 570mg	25%
Total Carbohydrate 38g	14%
Dietary Fiber 2g	5%
Total Sugars 11g	
Includes 0g Added Sugars	0%
Protein 8g	16%

Not a significant source of vitamin D, calcium, iron, and potassium

*The % Daily Value (DV) tells you how much a nutrient in a serving of food contributes to a daily diet. 2,000 calories a day is used for general nutrition advice.

Cinnamon Rolls Supreme

Yum.

1 Amy's Delicious Dinner Rolls recipe (see page 206)
fat-free butter spray
2 cups brown sugar
2 tablespoons cinnamon

Make the dough for rolls according to the recipe on page 190. After the dough has risen for the first time, punch down and put onto countertop. Roll out with a rolling pin until the dough is about 18 inches square. (It won't be a perfect square—just get it spread out in a square-ish shape!)

Lightly spray the entire surface of the dough with butter spray. You'll use about 20 pumps of the spray.

Stir the brown sugar and the cinnamon together in a bowl. Distribute this mixture evenly over the top of the dough. Spread with your fingers to smooth over the surface.

Roll the dough into a log shape. Use a very sharp knife to cut into 12 slices. Place the rolls in a 9x13 baking pan that you've lightly coated with baking spray. The edges of the rolls will be touching.

Cover with a clean cloth and set in a warm place to rise for about 40 minutes.

Bake at 375 degrees for 15 minutes or a until the tops of the rolls are golden and the cinnamon sugar is bubbly. Let cool for a few minutes before you dig in—you don't want to burn your mouth!

Serves: 12
Total Fat Content Per Serving (1 roll): 1 gram

Nutrition Facts

12 servings per container

Serving size	1 Roll

Amount Per Serving

Calories	360

	% Daily Value*
Total Fat 1g	1%
Saturated Fat 0.18g	1%
Trans Fat 0g	
Cholesterol 0mg	0%
Sodium 540mg	23%
Total Carbohydrate 79g	29%
Dietary Fiber 2g	9%
Total Sugars 36g	
Includes 0g Added Sugars	0%
Protein 7g	14%

Not a significant source of vitamin D, calcium, iron, and potassium

* The % Daily Value (DV) tells you how much a nutrient in a serving of food contributes to a daily diet. 2,000 calories a day is used for general nutrition advice.

Creamy Cucumbers

Fresh and cool for summer—take these to a July 4 party!

2 cucumbers, thinly sliced
1 small onion, thinly sliced
1/2 cup fat-free sour cream
1 tablespoon vinegar
1 teaspoon sugar

How's this for short and sweet? Stir together all the ingredients in a bowl. Cover and chill for at least one hour. Serve cold.

Serves: 4
Total Fat Content Per Serving: trace amounts only

Nutrition Facts

4 servings per container

Serving size	1/4 Recipe

Amount Per Serving

Calories	45

	% Daily Value*
Total Fat 0g	0%
Saturated Fat 0g	0%
Trans Fat 0g	
Cholesterol 0mg	0%
Sodium 25mg	1%
Total Carbohydrate 8g	3%
Dietary Fiber < 1g	3%
Total Sugars 5g	
Includes 0g Added Sugars	0%
Protein 2g	3%

Not a significant source of vitamin D, calcium, iron, and potassium

*The % Daily Value (DV) tells you how much a nutrient in a serving of food contributes to a daily diet. 2,000 calories a day is used for general nutrition advice.

Dude, You Don't Have to be Fat

Gourmet Grilled Cheese Squares

When you feel like highbrowing a lowbrow snack—or just cuz you like cheese as much as I do— this little ditty'll do the trick.

1 ¼ cups Kraft Natural Shredded Fat Free Cheddar Cheese
1 ¼ cups Kraft Natural Shredded Fat Free Mozzarella Cheese
     (or Lifetime brand of Fat Free Mozzarella Cheese, shredded)
1 tablespoon reduced-fat parmesan cheese
2 teaspoons minced garlic
1/3 cup diced green onions
Fat-free butter spray
10 slices sourdough bread
20 cherry tomatoes

In a bowl, mix cheddar cheese, mozzarella cheese, parmesan cheese, garlic, and green onions to make the gourmet cheese filling.

Spray one side of a slice of sourdough bread lightly with butter spray (about 5 pumps), and place it face down in a skillet. Place about 1/2 cup of the cheese filling on top of the bread, and sandwich it with a second slice of sourdough. Lightly spray the outside of the top slice with butter spray as well.

Cook over medium heat until cheese starts to melt together, then flip over in the pan. Continue cooking, flipping occasionally, until cheese is melted and both sides of the bread are light brown. Repeat to make a total of five sandwiches.

Cut each sandwich into four equal squares (for a total of 20 squares). Skewer a cherry tomato onto each square with a festive toothpick. Platter it all and serve at a party.

Note: If fat-free mozzarella is inexplicably hard to find in your area, substitute 2/3 cup of low-moisture, part-skim mozzarella instead. This adds about 0.5 grams of fat to each serving, which will still be fine.

Serves: 20 squares
Total Fat Content Per Serving (1 square): trace amounts only

Nutrition Facts

20 servings per container

Serving size	**1 Square**

Amount Per Serving

Calories	**100**

	% Daily Value*
Total Fat 0g	**1%**
Saturated Fat 0g	0%
Trans Fat 0g	
Cholesterol < 5mg	**1%**
Sodium 340mg	**15%**
Total Carbohydrate 16g	**6%**
Dietary Fiber 1g	4%
Total Sugars 1g	
Includes 0g Added Sugars	0%
Protein 9g	**18%**

Not a significant source of vitamin D, calcium, iron, and potassium

*The % Daily Value (DV) tells you how much a nutrient in a serving of food contributes to a daily diet. 2,000 calories a day is used for general nutrition advice.

Pizza Dip with Sourdough Chunks

The first time we had this at a BBQ it was all gone before we even got the meat on the grill. It's great to take to a party—or to enjoy as a snack for your own family.

1/2 cup Kraft Natural Shredded Fat Free Cheddar Cheese
1 block (8 oz) fat free cream cheese
1/2 cup fat-free sour cream
1 teaspoon oregano
1/8 teaspoon garlic powder
1/8 teaspoon red pepper (optional)
1/2 cup Hunt's Garlic & Herb Spaghetti Sauce
1/2 cup Hormel Turkey Pepperoni Minis
1/4 cup chopped green onions
1/2 cup chopped green peppers (optional)
1 loaf bakery-fresh sourdough bread

Mix cream cheese, sour cream, garlic, oregano and pepper. Spread into pie plate. Cover with spaghetti sauce, then other toppings. Bake 15 minutes at 350. Serve with sourdough bread torn into dippable chunks.

Note: You can add any other low-fat pizza toppings you like as well, such as pineapple, tomatoes, mushrooms, and so on.

Serves: 8 (about 4 dips per serving)
Total Fat Content Per Serving: 2 grams

Nutrition Facts

8 servings per container

Serving size	4 Dips

Amount Per Serving

Calories	250

	% Daily Value*
Total Fat 2g	3%
Saturated Fat 0.75g	4%
Trans Fat 0g	
Cholesterol 30mg	9%
Sodium 1020mg	44%
Total Carbohydrate 33g	12%
Dietary Fiber 1g	4%
Total Sugars 3g	
Includes 0g Added Sugars	0%
Protein 19g	38%

Not a significant source of vitamin D, calcium, iron, and potassium

*The % Daily Value (DV) tells you how much a nutrient in a serving of food contributes to a daily diet. 2,000 calories a day is used for general nutrition advice.

Dude, You Don't Have to be Fat

Rice Krispies® Treats Skinny-Style

Just cuz you're still a kid inside...

5 cups Rice Krispies brand dry cereal
4 cups miniature marshmallows
fat-free, non-stick cooking spray

Coat a glass bowl with non-stick cooking spray (about a 1-2 second spray). Microwave marshmallows on high for 2 minutes in the bowl. Stir, and heat in microwave for up to 1 minute more, or until marshmallows are fully melted. Stir until smooth.

Add Rice Krispies cereal, stirring to make sure cereal is well-coated with the marshmallow mixture.

Coat a 9x13 pan lightly with fat-free, non-stick cooking spray, and also lightly spray a spatula. Press the marshmallow mixture evenly into the pan and let cool. When ready, cut into 2-inch squares and serve!

Note: Because this recipe uses more than a quick pump of the non-stick cooking spray, it actually contains trace amounts of fat in the spray. So, while you want to use enough spray to facilitate the recipe, don't overdo it.

Serves: 24
Total Fat Content Per Serving (1 square): 0 grams

Nutrition Facts

24 servings per container

Serving size	1 Square

Amount Per Serving

Calories	150

	% Daily Value*
Total Fat 0g	0%
Saturated Fat 0g	0%
Trans Fat 0g	
Cholesterol 0mg	0%
Sodium 95mg	4%
Total Carbohydrate 37g	13%
Dietary Fiber 0g	0%
Total Sugars 23g	
Includes 0g Added Sugars	0%
Protein 2g	4%

Not a significant source of vitamin D, calcium, iron, and potassium

* The % Daily Value (DV) tells you how much a nutrient in a serving of food contributes to a daily diet. 2,000 calories a day is used for general nutrition advice.

Southwestern Snack Rolls

This is a nice cool snack for summer, and also an easy one to make-n-take for social gatherings.

1 block (8 ounces) fat-free cream cheese
12 ounces Picante sauce (about half a bottle)
8 fat-free or low-fat flour tortillas

Use an electric mixer to blend cream cheese and Picante sauce into a spread-able filling. Spread filling evenly on the tortillas. Roll the tortillas tightly, and then cut each one into six bite-sized snack slices. Spear each slice with a decorative toothpick, place on a plate and serve at your next party.

Note: You can use either mild or hot Picante sauce as suits your taste. Also, you can sub any other flavored salsa or sauce for the Picante sauce if you want to try variations on this simple, delicious snack.

Serves: 8 (six bite-sized snacks equals one serving)
Total Fat Content Per Serving: 2 grams

Nutrition Facts

8 servings per container

Serving size 6 Bite-Sized Pieces

Amount Per Serving

Calories 220

	% Daily Value*
Total Fat 2g	3%
Saturated Fat 0.5g	3%
Trans Fat 0g	
Cholesterol < 5mg	2%
Sodium 1030mg	45%
Total Carbohydrate 40g	15%
Dietary Fiber 5g	18%
Total Sugars 6g	
Includes 0g Added Sugars	0%
Protein 9g	18%

Not a significant source of vitamin D, calcium, iron, and potassium

* The % Daily Value (DV) tells you how much a nutrient in a serving of food contributes to a daily diet. 2,000 calories a day is used for general nutrition advice.

Superstar Smoothie

You'll love the burst of flavor in this fruity smoothie. Or try other fruits to customize to your liking.

1 cup frozen cherries
½ cup fat-free vanilla yogurt
½ cup orange juice

Place all ingredients into a blender, and puree until smooth. Pour into a glass, add a straw if you like, and start sipping!

Note: You can adapt this with any kind of frozen fruit chunks. Frozen peaches, mangos, and berries are all easy to find at your grocery store. You can also use different flavors of fat-free yogurt based on your preferences as well.

Serves: 1
Total Fat Content Per Serving: trace amounts only

Nutrition Facts

1 servings per container

Serving size	1 Smoothie

Amount Per Serving

Calories	220

	% Daily Value*
Total Fat 0g	0%
Saturated Fat 0g	0%
Trans Fat 0g	
Cholesterol < 5mg	1%
Sodium 70mg	3%
Total Carbohydrate 47g	17%
Dietary Fiber 3g	11%
Total Sugars 37g	
Includes 0g Added Sugars	0%
Protein 7g	14%

Not a significant source of vitamin D, calcium, iron, and potassium

*The % Daily Value (DV) tells you how much a nutrient in a serving of food contributes to a daily diet. 2,000 calories a day is used for general nutrition advice.

End Notes

Introduction
1 Jim Gaffigan. *Beyond the Pale* audio CD, Track #16: "Eat Healthy." (New York, Comedy Central Records, 2006).

How to Use This Book
2 David Zinczenko. *The Abs Diet Ultimate Nutrition Handbook*. (New York: Rodale, 2007) 2.

3 Dr. Kim Bruno, interview by Nappaland Literary Agency staff, July 7, 2011

4 Dr. Kim Bruno, interview by Nappaland Literary Agency staff, July 7, 2011.

One: Why Eat Well?
5 Bob Greene. *The Best Life Diet*. (New York: Simon and Schuster, 2006) 18.

6 Michelle Crouch. "Get Hired, Not Fired." *Reader's Digest*, April 2011, 133.

7 "Body Weight a 'Heavy' Influence on Career Success." Society for Industrial and Organizational Psychology, Inc., *siop.org*, February 19, 2008. http://www.siop.org/Media/News/Weight_Bias.aspx

8 Michael Cambray. "Does Being Overweight Affect One's Job Hunting?" Natural News, *naturalnews.com*, April 28, 2008. http://www.naturalnews.com/023114.html.

9 Richard H. Carmona, MD, MPH., FACS. "The Obesity Crisis in America." Office of the Surgeon General, *surgeongeneral.gov*, July 16, 2003, http://www.surgeongeneral.gov/news/testimony/obesity07162003.htm.

10 Editorial Board. "Editorial: Food Pyramid Now a Plate. Wow." *SLToday.com*, June 6, 2011. http://www.stltoday.com/news/opinion/columns/the-platform/article_bb9bba89-0a38-58ef-862e-ecb3b2c05ddd.html

11 Mary Clare Jalonick. "Obesity Rates Still Rising." HuffPost Social News, *huffingtonpost.com*, July 7, 2011. http://www.huffingtonpost.com/2011/07/07/obesity-states-rates_n_892181.html?icid=maing-grid7|main5|dl3|sec1_lnk3|76185

12 U.S. Department of Agriculture and U.S. Department of Health and Human Services. *Dietary Guidelines for Americans, 2010. 7th Edition*, Washington, DC: U.S. Government Printing Office, December 2010. Pg. 10.

13 Mary Clare Jalonick. "Obesity Rates Still Rising." HuffPost Social News, *huffingtonpost.com*, July 7, 2011. http://www.huffingtonpost.com/2011/07/07/obesity-states-rates_n_892181.html?icid=maing-grid7|main5|dl3|sec1_lnk3|76185

14 Eduardo Porter. *The Price of Everything*. (New York: Portfolio/Penguin, 2011) 66.

Two: First Steps
15 U.S. Department of Agriculture and U.S. Department of Health and Human Services. *Dietary Guidelines for Americans, 2010. 7th Edition*, Washington, DC: U.S. Government Printing Office, December 2010. Pg. 24.

16 Joseph C. Piscatella. *Fat-Proof Your Child*. (New York: Workman Publishing, 1997) 103-104.

17 Dean Ornish, MD *Eat More, Weigh Less*. (New York: HarperPaperbacks, 1993) 20.

18 Joseph C. Piscatella. *Fat-Proof Your Child*. (New York: Workman Publishing, 1997) 103

19 Tom Venuto, "Calorie Calculators & Calorie Calculations." *Freedomfly.net* "The Fitness

Network." *Freedomfly.com*, 2010. Accessed July 8, 2011. http://www.freedomfly.net/Articles/Nutrition/nutrition14.htm

20 Note: For a more precise estimate of daily caloric needs, fitness experts like Tom Venuto also use what's known as the "Harris-Benedict Equation," which factors in height, weight, age, gender, and activity level when determining recommended calorie intake. If you know your "lean body mass" you can get even more precise figures from using the "Katch-McArdle Formula." These equations can be a little confusing for guys (like me) who aren't math nerds, but they're not too difficult if you pay attention. If you want to check them out for yourself, visit: http://www.freedomfly.net/Articles/Nutrition/nutrition14.htm

21 Dean Ornish, MD *Eat More, Weigh Less*. (New York: HarperPaperbacks, 1993) 31.

22 "Pass the Pork Rinds, Consumers Want the Fat," USA Today, *usatoday.com*, June 24, 2001, http://www.usatoday.com/news/healthscience/health/2001-06-24-healthier-fat.htm.

Three: Fight SMART

23 Jason Hook. *Muhammad Ali: The Greatest*. (Austin, TX: Raintree Steck-Vaughn Publishers, 2001) 26-31.

Four: Simplify Eating Decisions

24 Lynn Fischer. *Fabulous Fat-Free Cooking*. Emmaus, PA: Rodale Press, 1997) 1.

25 Joseph C. Piscatella. *Fat-Proof Your Child*. (New York: Workman Publishing, 1997) 103-104

26 Joseph C. Piscatella. *Fat-Proof Your Child*. (New York: Workman Publishing, 1997) 103-104.

27 Joseph C. Piscatella. *Fat-Proof Your Child*. (New York: Workman Publishing, 1997) 103-104.

28 Joseph C. Piscatella. *Fat-Proof Your Child*. (New York: Workman Publishing, 1997) 103-106.

29 Louis J. Aronne, MD *The Skinny on Losing Weight without Being Hungry*. (New York: Broadway Books, 2009) 25.

30 "Endocannabinoids: The Human Body's Marijuana-Like Chemicals That Make Fatty Foods Irresistible." HuffPost Food, *huffingtonpost.com*, July 5, 2011. http://www.huffingtonpost.com/2011/07/05/endocannabinoids-fatty-food_n_890444.html

31 Jackie Warner. *This is Why You're Fat*. (New York: Grand Central Lifestyle, 2010) 16-17.

32 Georgia James. "Junk Food Makes Healthy Men Infertile, Study Says." *HuffPost Lifestyle*, United Kingdom. October 18, 2011. http://www.huffingtonpost.co.uk/2011/10/18/junk-food-makes-healthy-men-infertile_n_1017479.html.

33 Georgia James. "Junk Food Makes Healthy Men Infertile, Study Says." *HuffPost Lifestyle*, United Kingdom. October 18, 2011. http://www.huffingtonpost.co.uk/2011/10/18/junk-food-makes-healthy-men-infertile_n_1017479.html.

34 Robert K. Cooper, PhD, with Leslie L. Cooper. *Low-Fat Living*. (Emmaus, PA: Rodale Press, 1996) 19.

Five: Make It Easy to Eat Well

35 Louis J. Aronne, MD. *The Skinny on Losing Weight without Being Hungry*. (New York: Broadway Books, 2009) 3-4.

36 Jackie Warner. *This is Why You're Fat*. (New York: Grand Central Lifestyle, 2010) 5.

Six: Act Out Love
37 Wayne A. Detzler. *New Testament Words in Today's Language*. (Wheaton, IL: Victor Books, 1986) 268.
38 *The Revell Bible Dictionary*. (Old Tappan, NJ: Fleming H. Revell Company, 1990) 27-28.
39 Robert K. Cooper, PhD with Leslie L. Cooper. *Low-Fat Living*. Emmaus, PA: Rodale Press, 1996) 24.
40 "Child Obesity Statistics in America 2011." *Buzzle.com*, March 28, 2011, http://www.buzzle.com/articles/child-obesity-statistics-in-america2011.html
41 Robert K. Cooper, PhD with Leslie L. Cooper. *Low-Fat Living*. Emmaus, PA: Rodale Press, 1996) 23.

Seven: Recruit Allies
42 Paige Greenfield. "Are Your Friends Making You Fat?" O, The Oprah Magazine, *oprah.com*. January 2010. http://www.oprah.com/health/Friends-and-Weight-Gain-Diet-Advice_1
43 Nanci Hellmich. "Friends Help Carry the Burden of Dieting." USA Today, *usatoday.com*. January 7, 2008. http://www.usatoday.com/news/health/weightloss/2008-01-06-weight-loss-friends_N.htm
44 David R. Hamilton, PhD "Are Healthy (And Unhealthy) Habits Contagious? Huffington Post, *huffingtonpost.com*. May 29, 2011. http://www.huffingtonpost.com/david-r-hamilton-phd/health-social-networks_b_867433.html
45 David R. Hamilton, PhD "Are Healthy (And Unhealthy) Habits Contagious? Huffington Post, *huffingtonpost.com*. May 29, 2011. http://www.huffingtonpost.com/david-r-hamilton-phd/health-social-networks_b_867433.html
46 Nanci Hellmich. "Friends Help Carry the Burden of Dieting." USA Today, *usatoday.com*. January 7, 2008. http://www.usatoday.com/news/health/weightloss/2008-01-06-weight-loss-friends_N.htm

Eight: Take Charge of Your Attitude
47 Mark Richardson. "2011 Bugatti Veyron Grand Sport: Here's what it's like to drive a $2-million beast." Wheels magazine online, *wheels.ca*, June 17, 2011. http://www.wheels.ca/columns/article/798194
48 Dr. Kim Bruno, interview by Nappaland Literary Agency staff, July 7, 2011
49 Thomas B. Costain. *The Three Edwards*. (Garden City, NY: Doubleday & Company, 1958) 177, 179-180.
50 Lisa Dorfman with Sandra J. Gordon. *The Reunion Diet*. (North Branch, MN: Sunrise River Press, 2010) 27.
51 Alfie Kohn. *Punished by Rewards*. (Boston: Houghton Mifflin, 1993) 39-40.

Nine: Pantry Power
52 David Zinczenko. *The Abs Diet Ultimate Nutrition Handbook*. (New York: Rodale, 2007) 6.
53 David Zinczenko. *The Abs Diet Ultimate Nutrition Handbook*. (New York: Rodale, 2007) 2.

54 Unless otherwise indicated, all Food Groups info is taken from U.S. Department of Agriculture and U.S. Department of Health and Human Services. *Dietary Guidelines for Americans, 2010. 7th Edition*, Washington, DC: U.S. Government Printing Office, December 2010.

55 American Heart Association. *Low-Fat, Low-Cholesterol Cookbook, Fourth Edition.* (New York: Clarkson Potter Publishers, 2008) 336.

Ten: Shopping for Proteins

56 Joseph C. Piscatella. *Fat-Proof Your Child.* (New York: Workman Publishing, 1997) 104.

57 American Heart Association. *Low-Fat, Low-Cholesterol Cookbook, Fourth Edition.* (New York: Clarkson Potter Publishers, 2008) 21.

58 *Cooking Light What to* Eat. (Des Moines, IA: Oxmoor House, 2010) 98, 90.

Eleven: Shopping for Dairy

59 "Dumbocracy." *Reader's Digest*, June/July 2011, 119.

60 John J. Kohut and Roland Sweet. *Dumb, Dumber, Dumbest.* (New York: Plume, 1996) 44.

61 "Dumbocracy." *Reader's Digest*, June/July 2011, 119

62 USDA. DG Tipsheet #7: "Build a Healthy Meal." June 2011. http://www.choosemyplate.gov/downloads/TenTips/DGTipsheet7BuildAHealthyMeal.pdf..

63 *Cooking Light What to Eat.* (Des Moines, IA: Oxmoor House, 2010) 140.

64 *Cooking Light What to Eat.* (Des Moines, IA: Oxmoor House, 2010) 134.

Twelve: Shopping for Grain-Based Foods

65 William Sears, MD and Martha Sears, R.N. *The Family Nutrition Book.* (Boston: Little, Brown and Company, 1999) 128.

66 William Sears, MD and Martha Sears, R.N. *The Family Nutrition Book.* (Boston: Little, Brown and Company, 1999) 139.

Thirteen: Shopping for Produce

67 William Sears, MD and Martha Sears, R.N. *The Family Nutrition Book.* (Boston: Little, Brown and Company, 1999) 146.

68 *Cooking Light What to Eat.* (Des Moines, IA: Oxmoor House, 2010) 30.

69 Rory Freedman and Kim Barnouin. *Skinny Bitch.* (Philadelphia, PA: Running Press, 2005) 81.

70 Molly Morgan, RD, CDN. *The Skinny Rules.* (Don Mills, Ontario, Canada: Harlequin, 2011) 78.

Fourteen: Sugar, Desserts, Alcohol, and Salt

71 Rory Freedman and Kim Barnouin. *Skinny Bitch.* (Philadelphia, PA: Running Press, 2005) 27-28.

72 Jackie Warner. *This is Why You're Fat.* (New York: Grand Central Lifestyle, 2010) 27.

73 Louis J. Aronne, MD. *The Skinny on Losing Weight without Being Hungry.* (New York: Broadway Books, 2009) 26-27.

74 David Zinczenko. *The Abs Diet Ultimate Nutrition Handbook.* (New York: Rodale, 2007) 5.

75 Dr. Kim Bruno, interview by Nappaland Literary Agency staff, July 7, 2011

76 *The Calorie King Calorie, Fat, and Carbohydrate Counter*, 2011 Edition. (Costa Mesa, CA: Family Health Publishers, 2011) 23.

77 David Zinczenko. *The Abs Diet Ultimate Nutrition Handbook*. (New York: Rodale, 2007) 56.

78 Louis J. Aronne, MD. *The Skinny on Losing Weight without Being Hungry*. (New York: Broadway Books, 2009) 94, 160.

79 "Salt Shockers Slideshow." WebMD, *webmd.com*, June 20,20011, http://www.webmd.com/diet/slideshow-salt-shockers.

80 "Diet and Lifestyle: Salt Research." Internet Health Library, *internethealthlibrary.com*, March 28, 2001, http://internethealthlibrary.com/DietandLifestyle/salt-health-danger-research.htm

81 Steven Sinatra, MD and James Punkre. *The Fast Food Diet*. (Hoboken, NJ: Wiley, 2006) 42.

Fifteen: King of the Kitchen!

82 Molly Morgan, RD, CDN. *The Skinny Rules*. (Don Mills, Ontario, Canada: Harlequin, 2011) 105.

Sixteen: Eating Fast Food

83 Julie Watson. "Move Over Funnel Cakes, Fried Kool-Aid is Here." Associated Press, *newson6.com*, June 22, 2011, http://www.newson6.com/story/14957709/move-over-funnel-cakes-fried-kool-aid-is-here.

84 Steven Sinatra, MD and James Punkre. *The Fast Food Diet*. (Hoboken, NJ: Wiley, 2006) 2, 213

85 Kenn Kihiu. "America's Unhealthiest Restaurants – Revealed." Health Central, *healthcentral.com*, March 25, 2009, http://www.healthcentral.com/diet-exercise/c/58426/64620/unhealthiest.

86 Molly Morgan, RD, CDN. *The Skinny Rules*. (Don Mills, Ontario, Canada: Harlequin, 2011) 102.

87 *The Special K Challenge and Beyond*. (San Francisco, CA: Weldon Owen, 2011) 60.

88 Steven Sinatra, MD and James Punkre. *The Fast Food Diet*. (Hoboken, NJ: Wiley, 2006) 3.

89 David Zinczenko. *The Abs Diet Ultimate Nutrition Handbook*. (New York: Rodale, 2007) 27.

90 David Zinczenko. *The Abs Diet Ultimate Nutrition Handbook*. (New York: Rodale, 2007) 27.

91 Dr. Kim Bruno, interview by Nappaland Literary Agency staff, July 7, 2011

Seventeen: Fine Dining

92 Molly Morgan, RD, CDN. *The Skinny Rules*. (Don Mills, Ontario, Canada: Harlequin, 2011) 165.

Eighteen: Eating Socially

Nineteen: And Now...

Charts, References, and Other Helpful Info

93 Adapted from Metropolitan Life Insurance Company. "Height/Weight Chart." Memorial Hospital, Towanda, Pennsylvania, memorialhospital.org , 2003, http://www.memorialhospital.org/Library/general/weight-HEIGHT_W.html.

94 Menu items and fat counts taken either from a restaurant's Website or from *The Calorie King Calorie, Fat, and Carbohydrate Counter*, 2011 Edition. (Costa Mesa, CA: Family Health Publishers, 2011).

95 Menu items and fat counts taken either from a restaurant's Website or from *The Calorie King Calorie, Fat, and Carbohydrate Counter*, 2011 Edition. (Costa Mesa, CA: Family Health Publishers, 2011).

Mini-Cookbook for Men

96 All Nutrition Facts calculations for the Mini-Cookbook for Men were made using the nutrition facts tool at Livestrong.org. You can use this helpful tool for your own recipes by registering at www.LiveStrong.org. It's free!

About the Authors

Mike Nappa

is a bestselling and award-winning author with more than a million copies of his books sold worldwide. He's been enjoying the *Dude, You Don't Have to be Fat* lifestyle for over a decade. Plus, his wife said he was the "catch of a lifetime." So, you know, he's got that going for him.

Learn more about Mike at: *www.Nappaland.com/MikeNappa*

Dr. Edwin Risenhoover

is a family practice physician with two decades of experience practicing medicine. He holds a Bachelor's degree in Physics from Baylor University, and a Medical Doctorate from Kansas University. Dr. Risenhoover completed his Family Medicine Residency training at University of Nebraska Medical Center, and is licensed in Colorado.

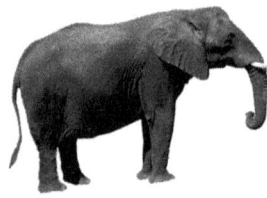

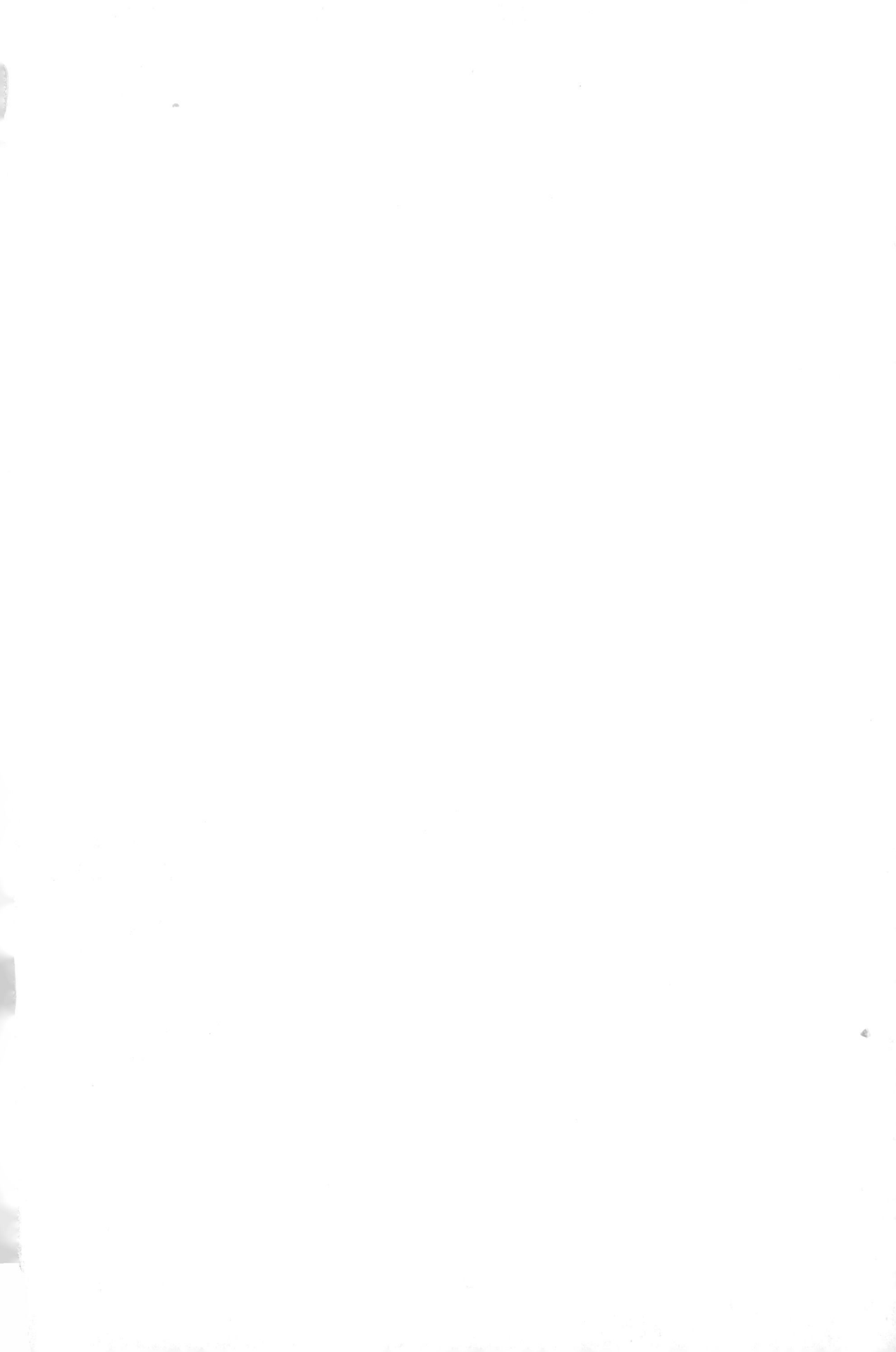

www.ingramcontent.com/pod-product-compliance
Lightning Source LLC
Chambersburg PA
CBHW080047280326
41934CB00014B/3246